STAFFORDSHIRE LIBRARY AND INFORMATION SERVICES
Please return or renew by the last date shown

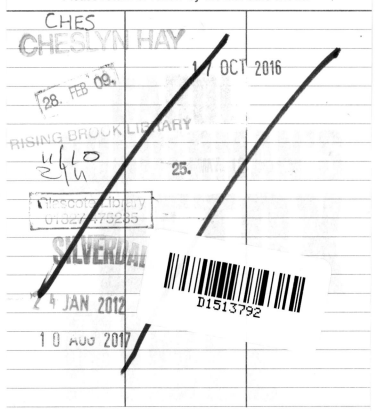

D1513792

If not required by other readers, this item may may be renewed
in person, by post or telephone, online or by email.
To renew, either the book or ticket are required

24 HOUR RENEWAL LINE 0845 33 00 740

CAROL VORDERMAN'S
mini
DETOX
BIBLE

From the million-copy bestselling detox plan

A complete detox for body and mind

with Anita Bean

Carol Vorderman
Sole Worldwide Representation

John Miles Organisation
Email: john@johnmiles.org.uk

Carol Vorderman was assisted in the writing of this book by Anita Bean BSc, one of the UK's most respected nutritionists and author and co-author of 17 best-selling books, including Carol Vorderman's Detox for Life series and Eat to Beat Cellulite. Winner of two major achievement awards in nutrition she is also a regular health writer for numerous magazines and a broadcaster on TV and radio.

CONTENTS

CHAPTER 1: **WHY DETOX NOW?** 7

CHAPTER 2: **TEN REASONS TO DETOX** 17

CHAPTER 3: **THE SCIENCE OF DETOX** 21

CHAPTER 4: **DETOX FOODS** 31

CHAPTER 5: **SEVENTEEN DETOX TIPS** 45

CHAPTER 6: **HOLISTIC DETOXING –**

MIND, BODY AND SOUL 55

CHAPTER 7: **DETOX YOUR LIFE** 65

CHAPTER 8: **DETOX – THE FUTURE** 75

CHAPTER 9: **THE DETOX PROGRAMME** 79

BREAKFAST 82

LUNCH 90

DINNER 108

INDEX 125

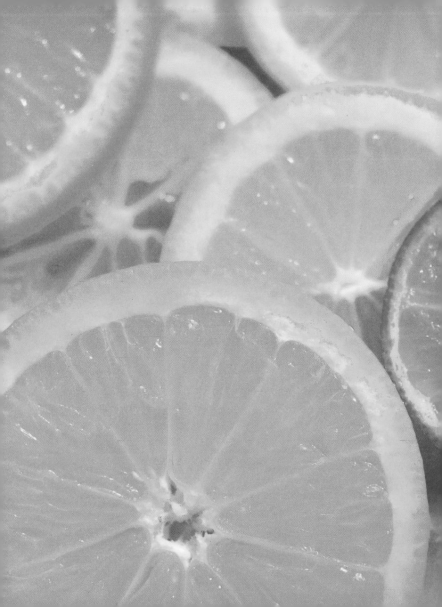

CHAPTER 1
WHY DETOX NOW?

In much the same way that you need a holiday, your body needs a break from its work. One way of restoring balance to the body is through a detox programme.

Everyone seems to have their own ideas about detoxing, ranging from a one-day fast and juice-only regimes to 'detox' pills, wearing 'detox' socks and having a 'detox' body wrap. All of these methods are without scientific foundation, and I certainly don't advocate any of them. Indeed, such products have no detoxing value and some may even do more harm than good, resulting in headaches and nausea.

I think of detoxing as a holistic lifestyle approach, rather than a quick fix. It stands up to scientific scrutiny that eating a healthier diet, taking more exercise and making better lifestyle choices reduce your exposure to pollutants and chemical toxins and strengthen your body's natural detoxifying systems, particularly the efficiency of the intestines, helping it, and other organs, remove toxins which are created metabolically in the rest of your system.

My detox diet programme, first published in 2001, was devised by Ko Chohan with nutritionist Anita Bean. It is essentially a vegetarian diet, with the emphasis on plant-based and unprocessed foods. This way of eating will help support your organs to efficiently release then remove the toxins from your system.

The result will be more energy, better sleep, reduced stress, clearer skin and an ability to manage your weight more easily. You'll lose excess weight gradually as your body finds its natural balance.

ARE YOU READY TO DETOX?

Toxin overload has a habit of creeping up on you. Tiredness, achy joints, weight gain and headaches are easy to ignore most of the time and are often put down to the stresses of everyday living. You may even regard them as a normal consequence of getting older. But they are often early warning signs that your body isn't processing foods as well as it ought to.

Poor eating habits can result in high intakes of dietary toxins, such as caffeine, alcohol and food additives. Stress and lack of physical activity make it harder for your body to process toxins and often trigger off food cravings and worse eating habits, setting up a vicious circle. What's more, if you smoke or take regular medications your poor body has an even bigger toxic load to deal with.

Air pollution, chemicals in the water supply, environmental pollutants (such as dioxins from pesticides, paints, varnishes and electrical equipment) and even the chemicals contained in household cleaners also increase your exposure to toxins.

The festive period around Christmas is, of course, a classic time for over-indulging in rich food and alcohol. Lack of sleep, stress, anxiety and lack of exercise all take their toll on your body. It's hardly surprising that many of us end up feeling sluggish and bloated in the New Year.

HEALTH AND DIET CHECK

When your system becomes overburdened with toxins, you develop a pattern of symptoms. One or two symptoms are probably no cause for concern. But when you develop a number of symptoms, that's when you need to take stock. Take the Health and Diet Check (in the following box) to find out whether you may be suffering from the symptoms of toxin overload.

This questionnaire is not intended to diagnose or treat any illness or underlying medical condition. You should always check with your doctor if you suspect you may have an allergy, infection or medical condition

HEALTH	YES/NO
I often feel run down, tired or lethargic	
I don't have much energy during the day	
I often feel irritable or get the 'blues'	
I seem to get one cold or infection after another	
I am prone to skin problems, e.g. acne, dryness, eczema	
My hair is dull or very dry	
My nails are very brittle or flaky	
I get a headache at least once a week	
I often feel bloated and suffer from indigestion or heartburn	
I often get constipated	
I often get diarrhoea or symptoms of IBS (irritable bowel syndrome)	
I have cellulite	

DIET CHECK	YES/NO
I have dieted on and off for several years	
I find it increasingly hard to lose weight and tend to put on weight readily	
I often eat when I'm not hungry	
I often skip breakfast	
I often snack instead of eating proper meals	
I don't eat five portions of fresh fruit and vegetables daily	
I eat the wrong foods when I'm bored, stressed or annoyed	
I drink soft drinks or fizzy drinks every day	
I eat sugary snacks (e.g. biscuits, chocolate, sweets, cakes) on most days	
I eat salted snacks (e.g. crisps, tortillas) on most days	
I eat fast food/ takeaways more than once a week	
I eat ready-meals at least twice a week	

YOUR ANSWERS

Your health

If you answered 'yes' to 8 or more statements in this section, this indicates your health is at risk. You will definitely benefit from detoxing. Minor health symptoms, such as those listed in the Health Check above, are often the result of poor eating habits and an inactive or stressful lifestyle. These conditions should not be ignored as they can be quite debilitating to your daily life and may develop into more serious complaints. It's clear that you need to take action straight away and look at ways of improving your lifestyle.

Eating more healthily, introducing more daily activity and taking steps to deal with stress are some of the ways you can improve your health and energy levels. Detoxing will help you regain your energy and restore your body's natural balance. Take action now!

Your diet

If you answered 'yes' to 8 or more statements in this section, this indicates you have poor eating habits that are almost certainly affecting your weight, your health and appearance. Your diet may be lacking in several important nutrients and you could be overloading your body with too much saturated fat, refined sugar and salt: all potential 'toxins' that can upset the normal balance of your body.

Eating an unbalanced diet with too many processed foods, too few fresh unprocessed foods and at erratic intervals during the day takes its toll on your energy levels and your health. Your poor digestive and elimination systems quickly become overburdened and result in bloating, indigestion and weight gain.

You need to take stock of your eating habits and make some simple changes to the way you eat. By opting for nutritious and mostly unprocessed foods, drinking more water and other hydrating fluids, and eating at regular intervals through the day you will quickly experience more energy and better appetite control. Detoxing helps you eat more in tune with your body's needs and teaches you how to control your appetite naturally. You'll find that you lose excess weight more easily and keep it off. Read on!

THE BENEFITS OF DETOXING

My detox programme is designed to restore your energy levels, improve your health and make you look and feel a lot better. It's not about calorie counting, strict dieting or measuring out tiny portions of food. It doesn't even require self-discipline, denial or restraint.

It's a healthy way of eating – based on ordinary foods – that fits in with your body's natural appetite and nutritional needs. You'll never feel hungry, you'll eat only the foods you like and you won't even need to spend much time cooking.

During the detox programme you will not only begin to feel healthier and happier but you will also experience gradual weight loss.

WHAT TO EXPECT?

Detoxing will improve the way you look, the way you feel and your ability to cope with stress. Like me, you may well find that you lose excess weight when you are detoxing because you will be eating healthier foods and feeling more positive about yourself. I dropped two dress sizes the first time I did the detox diet. Expect to lose up to 2½ kg (5 lb) in the first seven days (although some of this will be excess fluid) and then up to 1 kg (2 lb) a week. But you should regard weight loss as a natural consequence of the whole rebalancing process in your body. It's a sign that the detox programme is working well and your body is regaining its natural energy flow and rhythm.

HOW DOES THE DETOX DIET WORK?

The aim of this detox diet is to give your body a break from its usual toxin load by reducing the amount of toxins you take in and encouraging your body to eliminate old toxins.

More specifically, it involves:

● **Eating the right food to support the body's natural detoxification processes**

● **Opting for organic wherever possible (don't worry if you cannot always eat organic produce – eating the right types of food is more important)**

- Cutting out toxic substances such as nicotine, caffeine and alcohol

- Cutting down on foods and drinks that add to your toxin load – processed sugars, saturated fats, salty foods, additives

- Including certain supplements and herbs that support liver function and help detoxification

- Reducing emotional and physical stress in your life

- Adopting healthy habits such as exercise, relaxation therapies, better sleep and complementary therapies.

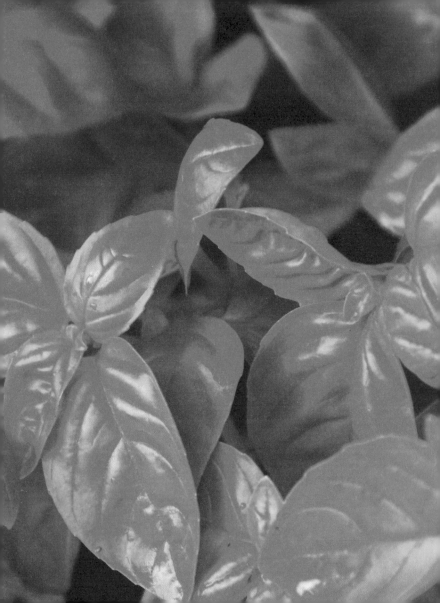

CHAPTER 2
TEN REASONS TO DETOX

1. WEIGHT LOSS

Cut out biscuits, takeaways and snacks, and eat instead whole grains, fruit, vegetables, beans, lentils and unsalted nuts. Fruit and vegetables are low in calories, virtually fat-free and filling. Satisfy your appetite with fibre-rich foods and you'll be less likely to turn to high calorie snacks.

2. CELLULITE REDUCTION

Lose fat and you lose cellulite – which 95% of women over 30 struggle with. A healthy diet with exercise and skincare are the only ways to beat cellulite.

Experts agree that ½–1kg (1–2lb) is a healthy and effective rate of weight loss in a week. And ½ kg of fat equates to roughly 3500 calories. So to lose ½ kg in a week you need to burn 3500 more

--->

-->

calories than you take in. This isn't as daunting as it sounds – lose 300 calories a day by foregoing a chocolate bar and step up your expenditure by 200 calories a day – equivalent to 40 minutes walking – and you'll lose ½ kg a week.

3. MORE ENERGY

By focusing on fruit, vegetables, salads, whole grains and pulses – foods that are fresh, have not been processed or overcooked and not adulterated with artificial additives – you'll provide your body with all the nutrients key to vitality and health. You'll reduce the toxin load on your system so you'll quickly begin to feel healthier and more energetic.

4. FEWER COLDS

By eating well, minor infections such as colds, sore throats and flu are less likely. Fruit and vegetables supply high levels of vitamin C, beta-carotene and other antioxidants in your diet and research shows that people with high intakes of these nutrients suffer fewer sick days.

5. LESS BLOATING

Swallowing too much air and eating in a rush are the most common causes of bloating. Chewing thoroughly and eating slowly helps reduce the amount of air swallowed with food. Avoid drinking fizzy drinks as they introduce more unwanted air. Try plain water and still juices. Bloating is sometimes a reaction to certain foods. Also cut out common bloating culprits such as yeast, wheat products and bran cereal.

6. LONGER LIFE

Numerous studies have linked a diet rich in fruit and vegetables with a lower risk of illness and diseases. One study found that eating at least five servings of fruit and vegetables each day could cut your risk of getting cancer by 20 per cent. Another found that people who ate the most fruit and vegetables had stronger bones.

7. LOWER BLOOD PRESSURE

The high content of potassium in fruit and vegetables helps regulate the body's fluid balance. A study found that 81 per cent of people with high blood pressure who started eating three to six servings of fruit and vegetables a day were able to reduce their medication by half.

8. SMOOTHER SKIN

Your skin rids the body of waste through sweating, skin oils and shedding dead cells. A study found that diets high in fresh produce give smoother and less lined skin than if you eat a lot of red meat and sugar.

9. SHINIER HAIR

The vitamins, minerals and phytonutrients (natural chemicals in plants that fight ageing and disease) in fruit and vegetables do wonders for your skin, hair and nails. A healthy diet improves the rate of hair growth, cell renewal and collagen formation.

10. SERENITY

Studies show that people whose diets are higher in fruit and vegetables find it easier to handle stress.

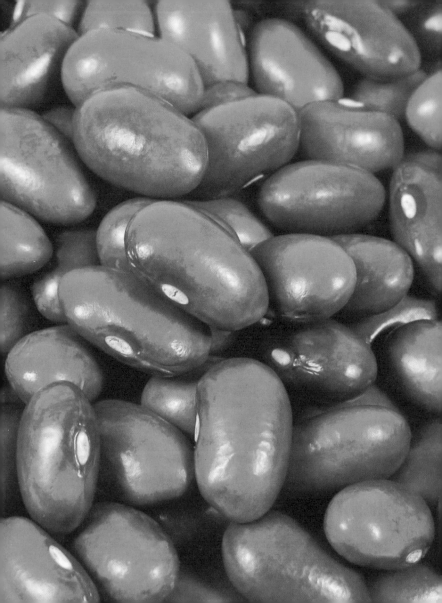

CHAPTER 3

THE SCIENCE OF DETOX

While the body is very good at detoxing itself, sometimes it can benefit from some extra support. A detox programme gives your body a break and helps it carry out its normal functions more effectively. For example, giving up alcohol eases the load on your liver; cutting back on caffeine reduces the stress on the nervous system.

The cornerstone of my detox programme is a low-toxin diet, plus plenty of vital nutrients needed to speed up the body's ability to detoxify. Doing this once (or twice) a year for a week, 14 days or 28 days, can make a major difference to your energy levels.

WHAT IS DETOXIFICATION?

Detoxification is the way your body gets rid of potentially harmful substances (toxins). It goes on all the time. Much of it is done by the liver, which transforms substances into something harmless or prepares them for elimination. In fact, your body is designed to cope with toxins.

The problem comes when you take in more toxins than your body can handle or your body's detoxifiers cannot carry out their job quite as well as they should. Your system becomes overloaded and you develop all sorts of symptoms, including bloating, lack of energy and dull skin. That's when you need to give your body a helping hand and it's time to embark on the detox diet.

WHAT ARE TOXINS?

Toxins are substances that are capable of harming your body. There are two main sources of toxins inside your body:

1. substances naturally produced in the body as a by-product of metabolism – every cell absorbs nutrients and oxygen and excretes wastes, like carbon dioxide;

2. substances that enter your body from the air you breathe; the food and drink you consume (e.g. pesticide residues, artificial additives, alcohol, caffeine, drugs and medications); or chemicals/pollutants absorbed through your lungs or skin from the outside world. These include pollutants in the air, cigarette smoke, exhaust fumes, detergents, household chemicals and toxic metals in the environment such as mercury and lead.

HOW THE BODY ELIMINATES TOXINS

Toxins have to be removed from the body and they leave through one of three exit routes: the bowel, the urinary tract or the lungs. The body also has 'emergency' exits to use if the main exits are sluggish: the skin and the mucous membranes. People whose exits are bottlenecked are more likely to have bowel problems, digestive problems, urinary tract infections, cystitis, recurrent swelling of the glands, catarrhal congestion and heavy periods. They are more likely to have skin problems and feel lethargic and run down as their liver struggles to cope with eliminating toxins.

YOUR BODY'S DETOXIFYING SYSTEM

Liver

This is your body's main processing plant. Its job is to make safe – detoxify – all potentially harmful substances. Once disarmed, these substances can then be eliminated via the kidneys, lungs or bowel. This work is carried out by thousands of enzymes. These enzymes require certain nutrients to help them do their job.

Kidneys

Their job is to filter out waste products such as urea (which is produced when proteins are broken down) from your blood into your urine. It's amazing to think that 7 litres (12 pints) of fluid pass through your kidneys every hour so it's important to drink plenty of water to dilute the toxins and help the kidneys carry out their job efficiently.

Gut

Your intestines not only process nutrients and toxins but propel indigestible material (mainly fibre) and potential toxins (from the bile) to the bowel. Fibre helps to mop up some of the toxins, stops them getting absorbed into your body and carries them to the bowel. Here they are disarmed by friendly bacteria and eliminated in the faeces.

Skin

This plays a big role in getting rid of toxins. Some toxins are eliminated in your sweat, others in your skin oils (sebum) and others via the shedding of dead skin cells.

Lymphatic circulation

This is like a drainage system. It carries waste products and potential toxins that are too large to enter your bloodstream from your cells to the lymph nodes for processing. They are then returned to the bloodstream and finally to the liver for detoxification.

Lungs

They filter out waste gases such as carbon dioxide that you produce in your body as well as toxic gases that you breathe in.

FOODS TO SUPPORT THE BODY'S DETOXIFIERS

The liver

Brussels sprouts, broccoli, cabbage, cauliflower, watercress and curly kale These vegetables are powerful detoxifiers, packed with nutrients that boost levels of an enzyme called glutathione. This enzyme helps the liver process toxic compounds and pesticides, which can then be safely eliminated in the urine and the stools. Glutathione is also a powerful antioxidant, protecting the liver from damage by processing toxins.

Garlic and onions The sulphur-containing compounds found in these vegetables boost levels of liver detoxifying enzymes.

Blueberries, blackberries, strawberries, raspberries These colourful fruits contain ellagic acid, which increases liver detoxifying enzymes, helping speed the removal of toxins.

Supplements Milk thistle, artichoke extract (silymarin and cynarin), garlic, dandelion, fennel.

The kidneys

Cranberries This fruit contains tannins that have unique 'anti-stick' properties. These stop bacteria adhering to the urinary tract walls and so help ward off infections. Fresh cranberries, unfortunately, are very sour but you can get all the benefits by drinking cranberry juice.

Celery A natural diuretic that also helps cleanse the kidneys.

Fennel Rich in potassium and flushes through the kidneys helping to eliminate toxins.

Supplements Dandelion, horsetail, cranberry, and celery seed.

The colon

Apples Rich in pectin, a soluble type of fibre that absorbs potential toxins and carcinogens from the small intestines and bowel, removing them via the stools.

Chickpeas Rich in fructo-oligosaccharides, which feed the 'good' bacteria in the gut, improve the balance of the gut flora, and speed the elimination of waste from the body.

Garlic Contains supernutrients that bind with toxins, bacteria and viruses in the body to render them harmless and promote their excretion.

Supplements Fibre supplements (psyllium), probiotic supplements, fructo-oligosaccharides, and aloe vera.

The skin

Pumpkin seeds and omega-rich oils (flax oil, walnut oil, pumpkinseed oil or blended essential oils) The high levels of omega-3 oils keep the cells in your skin watertight – if you don't get enough you risk dry, flaky, lifeless skin.

Mangoes and cantaloupe melon The high levels of beta-carotene in these fruits promote healthy new cells and boost the natural elasticity of the skin, creating smoother and more evenly textured skin even in cellulite-affected areas. The vitamin C in mangoes is good for strengthening collagen, the cement between skin cells.

Supplements Ginkgo biloba, essential fatty acid supplements (flax seed oil, evening primrose oil, fish oil), and antioxidant supplements.

The lungs

Oranges, blackberries, raspberries, peppers Rich in vitamin C, a powerful antioxidant that can protect against inhaled pollutants in the lungs.

Carrots, spinach, apricots Contain high levels of beta-carotene, which protects the lungs from free radicals in air pollution and cigarette smoke.

Supplements Antioxidant supplements containing vitamins C and E and beta-carotene

DETOX SUPPLEMENTS

It is not essential to supplement your diet while detoxing. The right supplements may, however, help your body's detoxifying systems work a little more efficiently and give your body an extra boost. The supplements below are readily available from health food stores, high street chemists and nutritional websites.

1. ANTIOXIDANTS

Antioxidants neutralise free radicals, which may otherwise harm body cells and even trigger off cancer and coronary artery disease. Free radical damage has also been linked to the ageing process and degenerative eye disease.

Antioxidant nutrients include various vitamins (including beta-carotene, vitamin C and vitamin E), minerals (such as selenium) and phytonutrients. They are found naturally in fruit and vegetables, seed oils, nuts, whole grains, beans and lentils. But, for extra protection, you can opt for a daily supplement containing several antioxidant nutrients.

Look for the following on the label:
Beta-carotene is a powerful free radical scavenger, destroys carcinogens (cancer causing substances), guards against heart disease and stroke and lowers cholesterol levels.

Vitamin C detoxifies many harmful substances and plays a key role in immunity. It increases a natural antiviral substance produced by the body and stimulates the activity of key immune cells.

Vitamin E is a powerful anti-oxidant that also improves oxygen utilisation, enhances your immune response and plays a role in prevention of cataracts caused by free radical damage.

Alpha lipoic acid is a potent antioxidant that promotes immunity and also helps protect the liver from alcohol damage.

Lycopene is a natural plant pigment, found naturally in tomatoes, that helps protect against prostate and lung cancer.

Lutein is found naturally in dark green leafy vegetables, protects against cataracts and is good for the heart, skin and eyes.

2. MILK THISTLE

This herb protects liver cells from effects of alcohol and other toxins. It contains silymarin, which helps the liver process toxins, stimulates the production of new liver cells and improves overall liver function.

It is also good for inflammatory bowel disorders, weakened immune system, and is beneficial for psoriasis and skin problems.

3. ESSENTIAL FATTY ACIDS

The omega-3 fatty acids found naturally in flaxseeds, walnuts and dark green leafy vegetables (as well as oily fish) improve oxygenation of your body cells, increase your energy levels and benefit your heart and cardiovascular health. They can also aid weight loss and boost immune function.

Taking a tablespoon of an omega-3 rich oil supplement will help boost your intake, especially if you do not consume oily fish. Many brands are based on fish oils, but if you prefer vegetarian sources, opt for a brand based on plant seed oils (e.g. flaxseed and pumpkinseed oils). Use in a salad dressing, on vegetables, whisked into soup, in smoothies or fruit juice or even porridge.

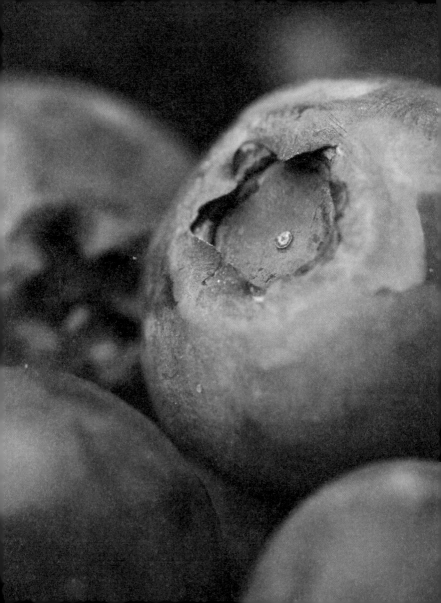

CHAPTER 4
DETOX FOODS

My detox programme centres on fresh, tasty and nutrient-packed foods that help your natural detox system work properly. It limits the amount of toxins you consume from heavily processed foods, artificial additives, caffeine, alcohol, salt and sugar, and so restores balance to your body.

WHAT TO EAT

Fruit and vegetables

Aim for five daily portions. All types can be included – ideally fresh but frozen varieties are also fine. Try to vary your choices as much as possible – don't stick with, say, apples and pears. It's a good idea to mix colours – yellow, green, orange, red, purple – as this will mean you'll get a good balance of vitamins, antioxidants and phytochemicals.

A high level of fruit and vegetables in your diet helps to boost your immunity and protect your body from cancer, heart disease and bowel disease. Eat fresh foods in season when they are less expensive and at their best.

All varieties of vegetables aid detoxification. Make at least one of your daily portions a cruciferous vegetable (broccoli, Brussels sprouts, cabbage, watercress, cauliflower). These contain glucosinolates, which boost the activity of your liver's detoxifying enzymes.

Vegetables are best eaten raw in salads or lightly steamed to get the most nutrients from them. To minimise vitamin losses, wash and prepare vegetables just before cooking them. Once they are cut, they start to lose vitamins. Put them straight into boiling water or steam them. Cook vegetables as lightly as possible: they should be firm and tender, not soft and soggy.

ORGANIC CHOICE

Choosing organic food will go a long way towards reducing your intake of toxins – pesticide residues, antibiotics, nitrates and hormones – but the price of organic food means that it isn't always realistic. If you can't eat organic all the time, concentrate on organic versions of salads and fruit, especially berries and soft fruit, as these foods are the most heavily sprayed and have the highest pesticide residue content. For other fruits and vegetables, wash them thoroughly in water or remove the peel.

Stir-frying is a good alternative to steaming or boiling as it preserves most of their nutrients and flavour.

Dried fruits (such as apricots, raisins, mango, figs) may be included –
they contain concentrated levels of fibre and many antioxidants, but are
also more concentrated in calories and (natural) sugars than the fresh
version, so eat them in moderate quantities only!

Grains, bread and pasta

Grains are rich in complex carbohydrates but opt for wholegrain
versions while detoxing. Wholegrains (such as wholegrain breads,
breakfast cereals, rice, oatmeal and millet) have a lower glycaemic index
(GI) than refined versions, which means they provide sustained energy
and satisfy your hunger longer.

They are also rich in fibre, B vitamins (especially thiamin and niacin),
vitamin E and minerals (such as iron).

Avoid wheat products (e.g. pasta, wheat-based breakfast cereals and
bread) while you are detoxing, especially if you are prone to bloating.
Many people find that replacing wheat with other types of wholegrains
– oats, brown rice, millet, quinoa – or other carbohydrate foods – sweet
potatoes or potatoes – for a short period helps reduce symptoms. After
detoxing, you can gradually reintroduce wheat.

Brown rice makes a delicious base for salads or fillings for vegetables
such as red peppers and aubergines. To save time, try the parboiled
variety, which takes only 10 minutes to cook.

Oats are also a good source of B vitamins, iron, magnesium and zinc. Use them in porridge, muesli or fruit crumbles.

Millet is a good source of magnesium and iron. Eat it boiled (like rice) or as a porridge, or add millet flakes to muesli and fruit crumbles.

Unlike wheat, rye contains no gluten so switching breads may reduce symptoms like bloating and wind if you are sensitive to gluten.

Quinoa (pronounced 'keenwa') looks like a grain but is, in fact, a fruit. It contains more protein than grains and makes a tasty alternative to rice or pasta.

Beans, lentils and peas

Include more beans, lentils and peas (collectively known as pulses) in your diet during your detox. These foods are packed with protein, complex carbohydrates, fibre, B vitamins, iron, zinc, manganese and magnesium.

Pulses are a healthy alternative to animal proteins (such as meat, poultry, and fish). The type of fibre found in these foods – soluble fibre – helps regulate blood glucose levels and makes you feel full longer. It also helps to lower blood cholesterol and prevent heart disease.

A word of caution, though. If you are not used to eating pulses, introduce them gradually to your diet, say 1 to 2 tablespoons, twice a week initially, increasing the amount and frequency over the coming weeks. This helps your digestive system adapt. Eating large amounts may cause wind, bloating, discomfort and diarrhoea. If you do suffer undue symptoms, cut back on the amount and build up gradually over a couple of weeks.

If cooking dried pulses, soak them overnight, drain and cook them in fresh water until they are soft (follow the instructions on the packet). Add a little salt-free vegetable bouillon, if you wish, but do not add salt until they have been cooked.

For convenience, buy tinned pulses. Drain and rinse if they have been tinned in salted water. Red kidney beans, chickpeas and flageolet beans are delicious in salads, adding texture as well as vital nutrients. Chickpeas are particularly good on a detox diet because of their high content of fructo-oligosaccharides, a type of fibre that increases the friendly bacteria of the gut.

Nuts and seeds

All kinds of nuts and seeds can be included in a detox diet. They are packed with important nutrients that help detoxification, benefit your health and reduce many of the symptoms of ageing and ill health. They supply heart-healthy monounsaturated oils and omega-3 oils, protein, fibre, B vitamins, iron, zinc and magnesium. Although they provide a lot of calories, these come mainly from essential fats, which help to lower blood cholesterol levels and protect against heart attacks.

Aim to consume one or two heaped tablespoons of nuts or seeds a day. Eat as snacks, sprinkled on salads or breakfast cereals.

Choose plain, unsalted nuts wherever possible and avoid those with coatings or flavourings.

For a nuttier flavour, try toasting nuts and seeds under a grill or in a hot oven for a few minutes.

Pumpkin seeds and linseeds (flax seeds) are particularly rich in the omega-3 oils, which are lacking in most people's diets. You'll need to grind linseeds in a coffee grinder to benefit from the oils, as they have a very tough outer husk. Add to muesli, yoghurt, shakes and smoothies.

When buying nuts and seeds, check the use-by date is several months away to ensure they are as fresh as possible. Store in an airtight container in a dark place, as they can quickly turn rancid if exposed to light and air.

Dairy produce and alternatives
Try to avoid cow's milk, cheese, butter and cream while detoxing and substitute non-dairy equivalents. Many people find that symptoms such as bloating, wind, nasal congestion or a runny nose improve once they

give their system a break from dairy products. You may gradually re-introduce these foods after 14 days.

Try rice milk, soya milk, almond milk or oat milk. Non-dairy milks contain healthier unsaturated oils (e.g. rapeseed) instead of saturated fats found in dairy products. Soya and almond milk are good choices as they provide good levels of protein and calcium.

You can also get protein and calcium from tofu (made from soya beans). As it doesn't have much taste on its own it benefits from marinating before using in recipes. Plain bio-yoghurt may be included in a detox diet as it is easier to digest than other dairy products and can usually be well tolerated by people with milk (lactose) intolerance. It is useful for boosting your protein, calcium and B vitamin intake during a detox.

Healthy oils

Seed and nut oils such as extra virgin olive oil, linseed (flax seed) oil, walnut oil, rapeseed oil and sesame oil are rich in the omega-3 fatty acids, which protect against heart disease.

Aim to include 1 level tablespoon a day. Don't fry with these oils, as high temperatures will reduce their nutritional value. Use olive oil for cooking and salad dressings. It is rich in monounsaturated fats and vitamin E. Choose extra-virgin olive oil rather than refined olive oil as it contains higher levels of antioxidants.

Try supplementing your diet with a tablespoon of an omega-3 rich oil supplement. Many brands are based on fish oils, but if you prefer vegetarian sources, opt for a brand based on plant seed oils (e.g. flaxseed and pumpkinseed oils). A mixture of these oils can be used in a salad dressing, on vegetables, whisked into soup, in smoothies or fruit juice or even porridge. Store in the fridge to stop them going rancid.

DETOX SNACKS

- A bowl of strawberries, raspberries, blueberries or blackberries
- A bunch of grapes
- A peach, nectarine or kiwi fruit
- A couple of plums or apricots
- A large slice of melon or pineapple
- A bowl of fresh fruit salad
- A banana
- Vegetable crudités with hummus or avocado dip
- A small handful of unsalted nuts (plain or toasted)
- A small handful of (unsulphured) dried fruit
- A small handful of seeds (plain or toasted)
- A glass of juice
- A smoothie

Herbs, spices and flavourings

Enhance the flavour of your food with herbs – such as basil, oregano, mint and parsley – lemon juice, lime juice, freshly ground black peppers, chilli, and cider and balsamic vinegar. Spices, such as coriander and ginger, are also good for detoxing as they help digestion.

WHAT TO AVOID

Wheat

Try to avoid or cut down on wheat while you are detoxing. This may help ease symptoms such as persistent bloating, digestive discomfort and flatulence. Many people are unaware they have a mild sensitivity to wheat protein (gluten) until they stop eating it. Cut out or cut down on bread, wheat-based cereals, ordinary pasta, white, brown and wholemeal (wheat) flour, ordinary noodles, cous cous, cakes and biscuits.

On the detox diet, without wheat you will find that your symptoms improve. You can then re-introduce wheat gradually and thereafter eat in moderation. However, if you suspect an allergy or intolerance to wheat, you should get a proper diagnosis from an allergy specialist and seek guidance from a doctor or dietitian.

Caffeine

Caffeine is a stimulant that mimics the effects of stress on the body. Coffee, tea and caffeine-containing soft drinks are often used as a quick-fix to boost flagging energy levels, increase your concentration or make you feel more alert. But the effect is short-lived. Drinking several cups of coffee throughout the day can leave you feeling more tired, irritable, restless and with a headache.

If you are used to drinking 6 or more cups of coffee or tea a day, don't give up overnight. This could lead to withdrawal symptoms, such as headaches. Cut down on caffeine gradually over a period of a week or two. Replace with water or herbal tea.

Alcohol

Try to avoid alcohol while you are detoxifying. The reason is that alcohol is a cell toxin. In the liver, it is broken down to acetaldehyde, which harms liver cells, the brain and muscles. It increases the production of harmful free radicals, destroys and uses up B vitamins and vitamins C and E. Alcohol acts like a diuretic, making your kidneys excrete more fluid and vital minerals (magnesium, calcium, potassium).

Salt

Do not add salt to any foods during cooking or at the table. Instead, flavour your food with spices, freshly ground black pepper, fresh herbs, lemon and lime juice, or cider vinegar. Avoid processed foods with high levels of salt: crisps and other salted snacks, ready meals, ready-made sauces, condiments, stock cubes, certain breakfast cereals, soups and foods canned in brine.

You get enough sodium (salt) from foods in their natural state. Fruit, vegetables and grains contain potassium, which helps rebalance the sodium in your body and flush out excess salt.

High salt intakes can cause fluid retention, bloating and dehydration. Over a period of time, excess salt can increase the risk of high blood pressure in people who are susceptible.

Dairy products

Try to avoid cow's milk, cheese, cream and butter while detoxing. If you are prone to a persistent stuffy or runny nose or congested sinuses, you may find symptoms improve. For some people, dairy products may create excess mucous in the sinuses and nasal passages. Other people find dairy products difficult to digest because of the lactose (milk sugar) content. This can cause bloating, discomfort and flatulence. Plain yoghurt (ideally bio yoghurt), goat's or sheep's milk products may be tolerated. Reintroduce dairy foods if you wish after you have completed your detox diet.

Meat and fish

Meat and fish are best avoided on the detox diet and substituted with other protein sources (see Beans, lentils and peas; Nuts and seeds; Non-dairy foods above). Concentrated forms of animal protein take longer to digest than plant protein so cutting them out for a while helps reduce the load on your digestive system – as well as reducing levels of saturated fats.

Avoid anything containing artificial sweeteners, colours, flavours and preservatives as far as possible. While food additives are judged by government committees to be safe to eat, they still add to the toxin burden on the body and their long-term safety is unknown. Check labels of ready meals, biscuits, cakes, desserts and spreads.

WHAT TO EAT CHECKLIST

- Fresh fruit
- Vegetables and Salad
- Unrefined non-wheat cereals – whole grain (brown) rice, oats, millet, quinoa, rye, buckwheat
- Non-wheat bread – rye bread, wheat-free, pumpernickel
- Non-wheat pasta – corn, millet or rice pasta
- Non-wheat crispbreads – rye, rice cakes, oatcakes
- Water, herbal or fruit tea, pure fruit juice
- Beans, lentils and peas
- Tofu and quorn
- Non-dairy milk – soya, rice, oat, almond or sesame 'milk'
- Nuts – almonds, cashews, hazelnuts, brazils, pecans, peanuts
- Seeds – pumpkin, sunflower, sesame, ground flaxseeds
- Extra-virgin olive, rapeseed, walnut, flaxseed or sesame oil
- Cold-pressed oil blends containing a mixture of omega-3 rich and omega-6 rich oils
- Fresh herbs

WHAT TO AVOID CHECKLIST

- Coffee, tea and other caffeine drinks (including decaffeinated drinks)
- Dairy products – milk, cheese, yoghurt, cream
- Sugar
- Cakes, biscuits, confectionery
- Meat
- Fish
- Eggs
- Wheat bread, pasta, noodles, crackers
- White rice
- Ready meals
- Salt
- Alcohol
- Artificial food additives
- Fried foods
- Artificial sweeteners
- Hydrogenated fats
- Fizzy drinks
- Squashes and cordials

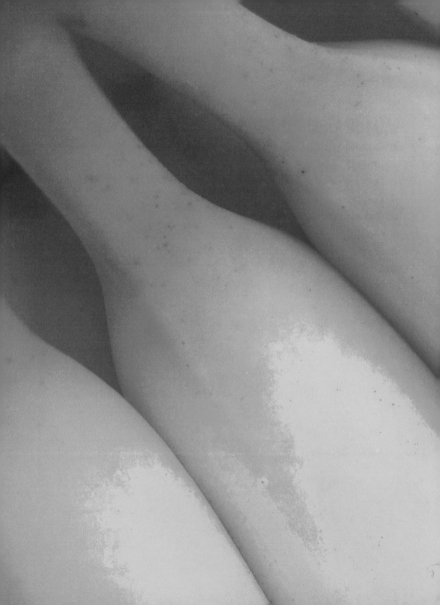

CHAPTER 5

SEVENTEEN DETOX TIPS

1. EAT FRESH FOOD

Eating fresh food means choosing foods that are rich in vital nutrients. As far as possible, try to buy fruit and vegetables that have been grown locally (not imported), that are in season and are not damaged or discoloured in any way. You may need to shop more than once a week as many fresh foods don't keep for more than a few days.

Food starts to lose its vitamins once it is exposed to air and light so store vegetables and soft fruits in a cool, dark place. Cut and prepare fruit and vegetables just before using them.

2. EAT RAW OR LIGHTLY COOKED FOOD

Uncooked fruit and vegetables contain the most vitamins. Once food is cooked, the vitamin content is reduced so try to eat them mostly raw or lightly cooked. That way, you'll be getting the maximum amount of vital nutrients. Certain foods (such as potatoes and dried beans and lentils) need to be cooked to break down the cell walls, soften the starch and make them digestible.

When you cook vegetables, try steaming them over a little boiling water so that they retain most of their vitamins. If you must boil your vegetables, use only a little water (about 1–2 cm) and add them to the pan only once the water has come to the boil. Cook them until they are only just tender, not soft and soggy. Some vegetables, such as mangetout, green beans or broccoli, taste better when they are still slightly crunchy.

3. CUT THE JUNK

Aim to cut out heavily processed foods from your diet. Foods such as biscuits, crisps and salty snacks, ready-made puddings and desserts, sweets, fizzy drinks and chocolate bars are practically devoid of vitamins, minerals and fibre. They are also packed with saturated fat, sugar, salt and artificial additives. By cutting the junk, you are reducing any toxic burden on your body.

Eating 'whole' and 'natural' foods provides valuable fibre that helps your digestive system work efficiently. You'll also get more vitamins, minerals and phytonutrients, plant substances that protect against illness and improve your all-round health.

4. GET A DRINKING HABIT

Make a habit of drinking water and other hydrating fluids regularly. Try to have a glass of water first thing in the morning and then plan frequent drinks during your day. Aim for 6 to 8 glasses (1 to 1½ litres) daily, more in hot weather or when you exercise. It's better to drink little and often rather than swigging large amounts in one go, which promotes urination and a greater loss of fluid.

Carry a bottle of water with you everywhere as a constant reminder to drink.

Many people confuse thirst with hunger. Both thirst and hunger sensations are generated at the same time to indicate the brain's needs.

If you don't recognise the sensation of thirst, you may assume that you are hungry, so you eat instead of drinking water. Next time you're feeling peckish drink a glass of water and wait ten minutes to see if you are still hungry.

WHAT TO DRINK

Not all of your daily fluid needs to be in the form of water. Count the following toward your daily fluid intake:

- **Fresh fruit juice, ideally diluted 1 part juice to 1 or 2 parts**
- **Home-made juices**
- **Herbal tea, e.g. peppermint, camomile, fennel**
- **Fruit tea**
- **Green tea**
- **Rooibos tea**
- **Clear homemade soup**

5. EAT WHEN YOU ARE HUNGRY

My detox programme is not a starvation diet. You should never go
hungry because it is based on fibre-rich nutritious food with maximum
filling power. If you feel peckish between meals, don't deny your hunger.
Instead, have a healthy snack – fresh fruit, a few nuts or seeds – and
don't feel guilty about eating.

Learn to listen to your body's hunger signals. This may take a bit of
practice as it can be difficult at first to work out whether it's food or drink
that your body really needs. Sometimes you may think you're hungry
due to boredom, stress or habit.

6. CHEW YOUR FOOD

Eating should be a pleasurable experience so make time to savour your
food.

Chew each mouthful of food carefully, as much as 30 times. Insalivate
it in your mouth and continue to chew before you swallow. This means
that the food is already half digested before it enters your stomach,
releasing a lot of stress on your stomach and intestines.

Try to focus on what you're eating rather than simply shovelling food into
your mouth and swallowing it. It's easier to notice you are full if you pay
attention while you are eating. It takes about twenty minutes before the
messages from your stomach hit your brain to say that you are being fed
and that you are full.

By chewing properly and eating slowly, placing your knife and fork down between mouthfuls, your body will be able to send a message to the appetite centres in your brain that it is satisfied, helping you to stop overeating. If you don't concentrate while you eat, your body may be telling you it's full but you may override the feeling of fullness and overeat.

Plan your meals for the whole week. Sit down with a pen and paper and work out exactly what you need at the supermarket. Making a shopping list before you go shopping means that you're more likely to stick to it, and planning ahead means you won't get home from work tired and hungry, only to discover there's nothing healthy in your fridge. Put all the non-detox foods in a separate cupboard so that you have just one cupboard where you go for your detox foods as well as the fridge. Make life as easy as possible for yourself.

Processed foods such as biscuits, cakes, chocolate and crisps are high in calories but lacking fibre, water and vital nutrients. They don't fill you up readily, nor do they satisfy your appetite. So your hunger signals become confused and you overeat. Eliminate these foods and eat instead lots of fibre-rich nutrient-packed foods – fruit, vegetables, whole grains and pulses – and your appetite quickly re-adjusts.

7. CHOOSE FIBRE-RICH FOODS

Eating more fibre-rich foods can help to reduce calorie intake. Fibre expands in the gut, makes you feel full and helps stop you overeating. It also helps to satisfy your hunger by slowing the rate that foods pass through your digestive system and stabilising blood sugar levels. Studies have shown that people who increased their fibre intake for four months ate fewer calories and lost an average of 2½ kg (5 lb) – with no dieting!

8. EAT REGULARLY

Eating smaller meals more frequently not only helps weight loss but also helps you recognise when you really are hungry. Spreading your meals more evenly through the day, as four to six small meals or snacks rather than two or three big ones, helps avoid blood sugar highs and lows and the resulting insulin surges. Have regular snacks of fruit, nuts or seeds to give you slow-release energy throughout the day.

9. PRACTICE PORTION CONTROL

It may sound obvious but larger portions make you eat more. A US study found that people ate 33% more food when given a large portion, even when they disliked the food. Try putting smaller portions of foods with a high calorie density (such as pasta, bread and nuts) on your plate and larger portions of low calorie energy density foods such as vegetables on your plate.

10. DON'T EAT TOO LATE AND ENJOY A GOOD BREAKFAST

If you eat too late it's like putting the accelerator down on your digestive system and then locking the car in the garage. Your digestive system has burnt out. When you're sleeping your body is trying to regenerate itself and this overload on your digestive system puts its natural processes out of balance. You will wake up tired and sluggish.

Ideally, eat little in the evenings, perhaps soup and steamed veg so that you wake up hungry and ready for a good breakfast. I have put recipes for lunch and dinner in the traditional way later in the book, but if at any time you can swap a light lunch with a heavier dinner, then do so. It will really benefit your detoxing and you will feel even better in the morning. You don't have to do this every day, I know how difficult that would be if you're working.

When you start your day off with a healthy filling breakfast, you dramatically increase your chances of eating healthily throughout the day. You also fuel your body and kick-start your metabolism, so you have the rest of the day to burn up those calories. If you don't eat breakfast, you're more likely to snack during the morning and overeat at lunch.

11. SLEEP MORE

Sleeping an extra hour or so may help you lose weight. A lack of sleep boosts levels of ghrelin, a hormone that makes you feel hungry, while lowering levels of another, leptin, that makes us feel full. This hormonal imbalance sends a signal to the brain that more food is needed, when, in fact, enough has been eaten. Research at the University of Chicago also shows that sleeping for four hours or less increases levels of another hormone, cortisol, which makes you feel hungry in the evening rather than sleepy.

12. SWITCH OFF THE TV

Don't eat in front of the television (nor as you're working or reading) as you don't notice what you're eating. Studies have shown that the distraction of TV postpones the point at which people stopped eating, such that they ate 12–15 % more. Also people who watch TV for more than four hours a day consume one third more calories because they have more opportunity to nibble (and less opportunity to exercise).

13. DISTINGUISH BETWEEN HUNGER AND APPETITE

Unfortunately, it is easy to confuse hunger and appetite. Appetite is produced by external stimuli such as the sight or smell of food or simply feeling bored. Real feelings of hunger are produced when your blood sugar begins to fall. The difference is that appetite goes away when you distract yourself with another activity. Next time you feel the urge to eat, distract yourself by going for a walk, taking a bath or doing your nails. If you're still hungry then you know you need to eat.

14. DON'T GO SHOPPING WHEN YOU'RE HUNGRY

If you go shopping when you're hungry you'll be tempted to fill up your trolley with high calorie foods. Make a shopping list before you hit the supermarket. That way you'll avoid unplanned supermarket splurges

in unhealthy foods. If you shop with a list you're less likely to make
impulsive food choices.

15. CARRY HEALTHY SNACKS

Always carry healthy snacks, such as apples, satsumas, nuts, or seeds
with you so you don't end up at the chocolate vending machine or
snack food counter when you're hit by hunger.

16. STOCK UP WITH HEALTHY FOODS

Keep a well-stocked supply of healthy foods that you love to make
your detox programme easy. Decide which new foods you're going to
substitute for high fat or sugary ones. This way, you'll keep yourself on
track and avoid the temptation of slipping back into old eating habits.
Remember, fruit, vegetables, pulses and wholegrain cereals give best
filling power for minimum calories. They contain lots of water and fibre,
which fill you up, slow down your eating speed and give best meal
satisfaction. Choose the ones you like and stock up on those.

17. DIY LUNCH

Bring your own lunch to work – you'll have more control over how
many calories you eat. A study found that people who eat in restaurants
daily consume 300 more calories a day than those who prepare their
own food. Try hummus with crudités and rye crackers or a pasta salad.

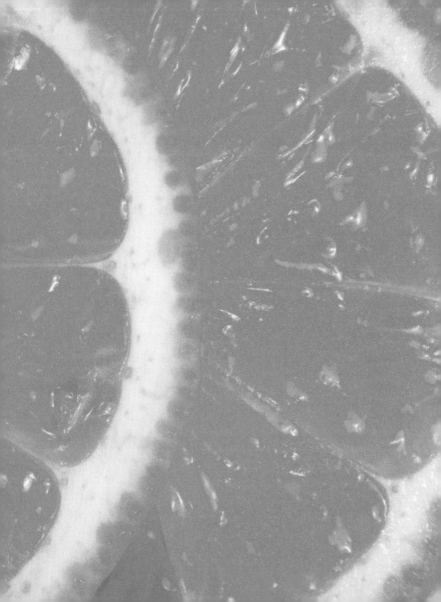

CHAPTER 6
HOLISTIC DETOXING — MIND, BODY AND SOUL

As well as eating a healthier diet, it is also important to detox on an emotional and psychological level. Unless you deal with it, the stress of living a hectic life can keep growing and eventually interfere with the body's healing ability.

On-going stress results in symptoms such as fatigue, sleep problems and poor health.

Every so often, you should put aside time to reassess, regain control and strengthen your mind, body and soul. A relaxed and positive state of mind can boost your immunity and well-being.

Developing a positive mental attitude, greater self-belief, more confidence, and gaining support from your family and friends all improve your chances of success fully achieving peak health.

STRESS-BUSTING TIPS

1. Try forms of exercise that offer mental as well as physical benefits e.g. yoga or t'ai chi.

2. Build into your schedule some time each day that is just for you to do exactly what you want.

3. Practise relaxation techniques and controlled breathing. When you're stressed your breathing becomes shallow. Deep breathing slows your heart rate, lowers your blood pressure and eases anxiety.

4. Accept that you cannot control everything. Control the things you can but learn to let go and delegate things to others – you'll find stress levels drop dramatically.

5. Learn to prioritise. Make a list of jobs that need to be done, prioritise them and then allocate time for them in a diary.

6. Have fun – try to do what you love and love what you do.

EXERCISE

Regular exercise is good for every system in your body, in particular your heart and lungs. It also improves your detoxification systems, your mental wellbeing, influencing your ability to deal with stress and anxiety.

You are more likely to stick with an exercise programme if you enjoy it, so pick an activity that suits you. All types of exercise, from walking and gentle jogging to swimming and weight training can help alleviate stress and bring inner calm. As well, exercise helps promote a healthy digestive system and a lower resting heart rate. There are two main forms of exercise, although you are likely to find elements of more than one in any particular sport.

Aerobic exercise
This type of exercise includes any activity that increases your breathing and heart rate for an extended period: walking, running, hiking, swimming, cycling, rowing, and aerobic fitness classes. Aerobic exercise is good for your heart – the heart and lungs have to work harder than normal as well as burning body fat, relieving stress and stimulating the immune and lymphatic systems. For maximum benefit, aim for 20 to 60 minutes of low to moderate intensity exercise 3 to 5 times a week.

Anaerobic exercise
This type of exercise involves short intense bursts of activity, followed by rest periods: for example weight lifting, body pump, sprinting, rope skipping and press-ups. Many sports such as tennis, squash, hockey and football also include anaerobic movements. These activities improve your muscle tone, strength, speed and power. They can also help combat stress as well as boost your body image and confidence. For best results, you should include two sessions a week.

YOGA
The word yoga comes from Sanskrit, the language of ancient India, meaning 'union', describing the experience of integration or wholeness with your inner self.

The most common type practised in the West is hatha yoga, a combination of asanas (physical exercises and postures), pranayama (breathing techniques) and meditation. It works to achieve perfect physical and mental health, happiness and tranquillity. It also reconditions the nerve-muscle and nerve-gland systems enabling them to withstand high levels of stress.

Many people learn yoga by attending classes, although videos and books are also popular. As with all exercises, technique is very important and for this reason it's advisable for beginners to seek out a qualified teacher.

Yoga can be practised by anyone at any age. It develops flexibility and muscular endurance and incorporates techniques to relieve stress and bring the mind and body into harmony. Exercising at the beginning of the day can counteract morning stiffness and give you energy. Exercising in the evening can relax you and help promote sound refreshing sleep.

To find a teacher: The British Wheel of Yoga has a national network of over 3000 qualified teachers. Contact www.bwy.org.uk to find a local teacher.

BREATHING

Learning to breathe properly increases the oxygen flow to every cell in your body, helping the detoxification process. It will also relax you and relieve stress. Sit, stand or lie down. Relax your shoulders and hands. Place your fingertips on your stomach. Close your eyes and breathe in slowly, counting to four. Feel your chest expand as the air fills your lungs. Hold for a count of four and then slowly breathe out for another count of four. Before taking the next breath, pause for a few seconds. Repeat a few times and continue to focus your attention on your breathing. After this you will be feeling calmer and more relaxed.

MEDITATION

Meditation is a technique for calming a restless mind. You focus your attention on one thing to the exclusion of everything else. When the mind is quiet you feel peaceful. Meditating regularly helps to bring deep-seated tensions to the surface where you can examine them and deal with them. Once you confront and resolve issues you feel more at ease with yourself and experience greater confidence and sense of self-worth. People who practise regular meditation have fewer health complaints and a lower incidence of disease. It can also help treat disorders such as high blood pressure, migraine and heart disease. A simple meditation:

1. **Sit comfortably upright – try sitting on your heels, place your palms on your knees. Close your eyes and breathe regularly. Keep as relaxed as you can.**

2. **Inhale slowly and smoothly through your nose.**

3. **As you breathe out slowly and smoothly mentally say the word 'one'.***

4. Repeat steps 2 and 3 several times. Keep your breathing slow and smooth. If your thoughts wander, gently guide them back to your breathing and repetition of the word 'one' or your chosen phrase.

5. When you are ready to end your meditation, open your eyes gently and gently stretch your limbs.

* You may substitute any word or phrase for 'one'. Suggestions are 'peace', 'calm', 'love' or 'I am at peace'.

REFLEXOLOGY

Some people believe that the ancient practice of reflexology can be used for maintaining and restoring the body's natural balance. It claims to treat the whole person and not just the symptoms it is a great way of relaxing the body and mind and dealing with stress.

Reflexologists apply pressure to specific reflex points on the feet and hands. Each reflex point corresponds to a part of the body. By applying pressure to these points therapists claim to stimulate or rebalance energy to the related zone and trigger the body's own healing system. It can help the body expel toxins, release tension and restore its natural state of balance. Reflexology claims to treat stress, menstrual problems, fatigue, general aches and pains, eczema, earache and migraine as well as many other conditions.

To find a reflexologist: contact the Association of Reflexologists www.aor.org.uk.

AROMATHERAPY

The use of essential oils, extracted from the flowers, fruits, leaves, stems and roots of plants is good for stress-related conditions, insomnia and emotional problems.

Essential oils may be inhaled or absorbed through the skin. For inhalation, place one to five drops on a tissue or in a burner or vaporiser. Use them to scent rooms, enhance your mood and relieve stress.

Oils massaged into the skin pass into the bloodstream and can influence nervous system functions, resulting in calmness and relaxation. Dilute one to five drops of the oils per teaspoon (5 ml) of carrier oil, such as sweet almond or wheatgerm.

Try adding the oils to your bath. For best effect, add four to six drops to a teaspoon of carrier oil or milk and mix vigorously in the water. Some oils shouldn't be used if you're epileptic, have asthma or high blood pressure, or are pregnant.

To find a therapist: contact the Aromatherapy Consortium, Tel: 0870 774 3477, www.aromatherapy-regulation.org.uk.
For more information about essential oils and their uses: www.bbc.co.uk/health/healthy_living.

MASSAGE

Massage is great for promoting relaxation, healing and wellbeing. There are several different types but all combine the soothing properties of touch with the skilful manipulation of muscles, tendons and ligaments. Massage also improves the flow of blood and lymph fluid, helps to eliminate waste products from the body, and relaxes the muscles.

When the body is touched, receptors in the skin send messages to the brain causing the release of chemicals such as endorphins. These produce a sense of relaxation and wellbeing and can also relieve pain.

Oriental massage therapies are based on the 'meridian' system of energetic channels that course through the body. Pressure techniques are thought to release blockages and improve the flow of vital energy (or 'chi') in these channels.

Massage is also useful for specific ailments such as asthma, depression, neck and back pain, insomnia, and diabetes.

To find a therapist: Massage therapists can be found at most beauty clinics, health clubs, spa resorts and complementary medicine clinics. One of the most widely accepted general massage qualifications is the ITEC diploma. Alternatively, therapists may have diplomas in specific massage techniques such as reflexology, aromatherapy, shiatsu, or Indian head massage.

AYURVEDA

Ayurvedic medicine is the traditional medicine system of India. Ayurveda means 'science of life', the guiding principle is that the mind influences the body. Studies have shown it to be effective for many disorders including digestive, skin and gynaecological problems, nasal congestion, sluggish digestion and stress.

One of the key principles of ayurveda is that of the five elements (panchamahabhutas) – ether (akasha), air (vayu), fire (agni), water (jala) and earth (prithvi) – which combine to form three vital energies (doshas), known as vata, pitta and kapha, which make up your constitution.

Each dosha has its own characteristics. Typically one or two doshas will dominate and the balance between these doshas determines your individual constitution and predisposition to disease.

Ayurvedic treatment aims to restore the balance of the doshas. It typically starts by first detoxifying the body to eliminate disease or any blockages or imbalances in the body. During a consultation, you will be advised on your lifestyle, diet and exercise. Herbal medicines may be combined with massage and manipulation, and yoga exercises. According to ayurvedic medicine the best foods for you are those that suit your constitution.

To find a practitioner: Ayurvedic Medical Association UK, 1079 Garratt Lane, London SW17 0LN, Tel: 020 8682 3876 (no website), maintains the register of qualified ayurvedic practitioners.

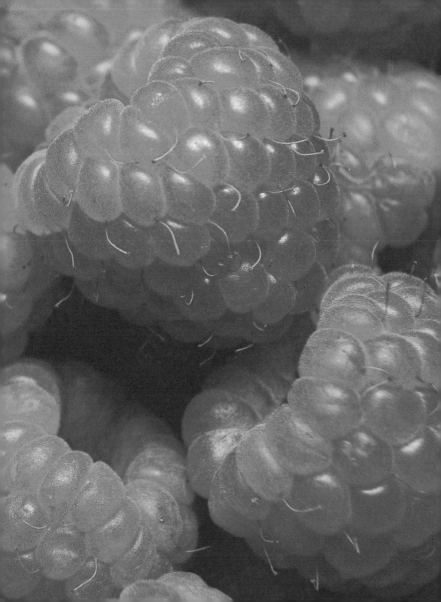

CHAPTER 7
DETOX YOUR LIFE

Unfortunately there are environmental toxins all around us, in the air, our water supply and our food. As well as detoxing your body by adjusting your diet, you should also try to reduce exposure to toxins and pollutants in your everyday life. Try to follow as many of the following steps as you can.

GO ORGANIC

There are strict limits on the levels of pesticide residues, antibiotics, nitrates and hormone residues allowed in food but choosing organic will help keep your intake of toxins as low as possible.

The high price of organic food means that it isn't always realistic. If you can't eat organic all the time, just concentrate on organic versions of salads and fruit, especially berries and soft fruit, as these foods are the most heavily sprayed and have the highest pesticide residue content. Wash non-organic fruit and vegetables thoroughly in water to help remove residues.

Buying organic also reduces the potential long-term risk of additives. Organic processed foods have a strictly controlled list of permitted additives.

AVOID DIOXINS

Dioxins are common pollutants – produced as the result of many industrial processes, as well as paints, varnishes, electrical equipment and flame-retardants. They can get into our water systems and soil and end up in the food we eat.

They have been found in breast milk, and can cross the placenta between mother and unborn child. Doctors believe that exposure to low levels of these chemicals during critical periods of development can have harmful effects, particularly involving fertility – but this is hard to prove in humans, and they do not know why it happens.
Dioxins are found mostly in fat-rich foods, such as meat, full fat dairy products and oily fish. Many of these are not included in the detox programme but when you begin your maintenance programme, opt for skimmed dairy products, lean meat and eat oily fish such as salmon once or twice a week.

LESS PLASTIC

It's difficult to escape from plastics – they are found in packaging, appliances and food containers. The problem is they contain petroleum or oil and other chemicals, which are capable of being leached out into the air, food or water. Toxins from plastic food packaging and containers (especially pvc), for example, can leach and transfer to the food that they come into contact with. These plastic toxins may interfere with hormones in the body, and have been blamed for early puberty, birth defects and infertility.

HOW TO CUT YOUR RISK FROM PLASTICS

Cut your risk by switching from plastic food containers to containers made out of other materials such as glass, ceramics or non-reactive metals.

Try to buy foods not wrapped in plastic packaging as far as possible (although this can be hard to avoid).

Never heat food in plastic containers or in contact with plastic films – they leak out even more toxic chemicals into the food.

Avoid direct contact of foods with plastic film by keeping food in glass or ceramic containers with the film stretched over the top.

Replace vinyl with non-toxic materials like linoleum, slate, quarry tiles, cork or wood.

CUT DOWN EXPOSURE TO AIR POLLUTION

Avoid walking in traffic-dense areas in cities and use side streets rather than main roads wherever possible.

Traffic produces harmful pollutants, which are especially harmful for people with breathing problems, lung conditions and asthma. The main culprits are nitrogen dioxide and sulphur dioxide (which combines with oxygen and water to form sulphuric acid), ozone (which is formed when polluting chemicals react in sunlight) and particulates (the large molecules thrown out in diesel fumes).

On hot humid days you can even see the nitrogen dioxide on the sky as a brown haze over the horizon.

These chemical pollutants irritate our airways, from the throat right down to the tiny passageways deep in our lungs. This is particularly bad news for people with asthma but it's not good news even if you are fit. According to a study in the medical journal *Thorax*, exposure to these pollutants reduces breathing capacity in both healthy and asthmatic people by up to 10 per cent.

SWITCH TO NON-TOXIC HOUSEHOLD CLEANING PRODUCTS

Switching to safe non-toxic cleaning products is an easy way to reduce the amount of pollution in your home. Toxic chemicals are found in window cleaning products, carpet cleaners, chlorine and bleach-based cleaners, metal polishes and oven cleaners.

These toxins may cause a variety of symptoms, including migraines, respiratory problems, rashes, fatigue and eye irritation. The connection may not be immediately apparent but you can cut your risks by tossing out your chemical-based products and buy 'green' cleansers, which contain non-petroleum based surfactants, are chlorine- and phosphate-free, claim to be non-toxic and are biodegradable. There are a number of good brands of household cleaning products that are safe and effective. The good ones list the ingredients, the risky ones won't.

Go back to tried and tested methods

Clean sinks with hot water and bicarbonate of soda or use vinegar to clean windows.

Oven cleaners contain highly toxic chemicals. Try 'green' versions or putting a drip pan in the bottom of your oven and wipe up spills as soon as they happen before they become hardened and baked on. You can usually clean appliances like your oven with just some water, soap and a bit of elbow grease.

Many people are obsessed with over-zealous hygiene and believe antibacterial cleaners are necessary to kill every bug. But some doctors believe that bringing up our children in scrubbed disinfected modern houses may result in their immune system becoming oversensitive. Later, when exposed to germs and potential allergens they are more likely to become allergic to them. Research suggests that antibacterial additives in washing up liquids and other cleansers aren't necessary.

REDUCE CHLORINE EXPOSURE

Chlorine is an ingredient in bleach, and a potential toxin. It is found in many household products including toilet cleaners, surface cleaners and certain laundry products. When heated, chlorine gives off organochlorines, which are highly carcinogenic.

Instead of using chlorine-or bleach-based cleaners try more natural or environmentally friendly cleansers. There are several brands of toxin-free cleansers. As a safe alternative to toilet descalers, use baking soda or vinegar and leave in the toilet overnight.

Try switching to unbleached tissues and toilet tissues, paper towels, coffee filters. Use a water filter to remove chlorine from tap water or use bottled mineral water instead.

AN ORGANIC GARDEN

Garden chemicals – fertilisers, insecticides – can potentially damage the immune system. Use organic and natural alternatives, which are widely available at garden centres.

DETOX YOUR HOME

While detoxing your body you may find it helpful to simplify your surroundings. Just changing the position of certain items and using colour wisely can improve the flow of energy in your home, and have a therapeutic effect on many aspects of your life, including your health and happiness.

Surrounding yourself with clean, clear surfaces can help you feel more relaxed. There's nothing more energy sapping than living in a muddle or mess. Decluttering and lightening your load at home will clear your mind and focus your energies.

Managing your space

● **Clear out the clutter – carefully consider what ornaments, furniture, books, etc. are really necessary and get rid of stuff you don't really need**

● **Recycle old magazines and books**

● **Go through cupboards and drawers one at a time, throwing out accumulated rubbish and retaining only what is strictly necessary**

● Clear all work surfaces at the end of each day

● Donate any clothing you haven't worn for 12 months to charity

● Visit the local dump about twice a year to get rid of bulky objects that are no longer needed

● Rearrange the furniture – experiment with new circulation routes and break the grip of habit in your surroundings

● Make a peaceful home

● Letting more light into your home, changing colours and shades can dramatically change the way you feel.

Light, shade and colour

● Use mirrors to maximise the flow of energising natural light through your home. Light promotes physical vitality and mental alertness.

● Use sheer fabrics for curtains or shades to diffuse and soften the light where appropriate e.g. in living rooms or dining rooms

● Choose flexible artificial lighting – try a number of alternative light sources at different heights in a room, including table lights, directional lights for work or reading, picture lighting and some upward lighting to create an ambient mood

● Use candles to create mood lighting. Try burning aromatherapy candles or floating candles in decorative bowls filled with water to establish ambience. (Never leave candles unattended.)

- Use colours strategically to create different moods. Cooler colours tend to be calming, warmer hues stimulating

- Natural textures and materials such as slate, cotton, wood and hessian contribute to a restful atmosphere

- Use cushions in different colours to add changeable accents of colour to suit your mood.

The feel-good home

- Fresh flowers in a house are lovely

- Use aromatherapy oils to scent your rooms with a relaxing fragrance

- Put houseplants around your home and office – household plants such as palms, chrysanthemums and ferns help reduce chemical levels in the atmosphere

- Place something in your entrance hall, or by your front door, to remind you to unwind when you come home. This could be a plant, a plaque or an ornament

- Have an aquarium – fish can be very soothing to watch

- Make the hearth a focal point of the room (instead of the TV) – this creates homeliness – and add candles and photos to your hearth. Make a real fire, only if you have a fully operational chimney, of course.

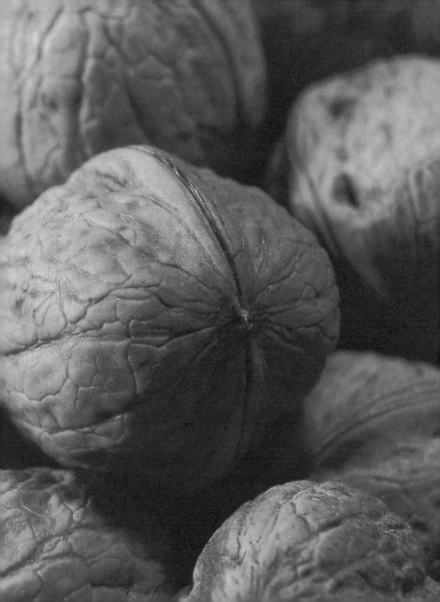

CHAPTER 8
DETOX – THE FUTURE

My detox programme will re-energise and rebalance your body. But it will also re-educate your palate so you learn to prefer healthier foods long term. You should adapt the principles of the detox diet to your future diet.

HOW OFTEN?

No one is perfect and sometimes it is easy to let good habits slide. For example, during stressful periods, on holiday or during the Christmas festivities, you may not eat as healthily as usual. Toxins may begin to accumulate and your system gets overworked again. You will start to recognise those symptoms of toxin build-up.

That's the time to take stock and go back on the detox diet. You may need to do this once every 6 months or once a year; for example, in the New Year, or during the spring and early summer months. When we have more exposure to sunlight, the brain releases the feel good chemical serotonin, which lifts our mood and makes the detox process easier by naturally reducing appetite.

It may not always be necessary to do the full detox. You may feel that a partial detox, say cutting out alcohol, caffeine, and heavily processed foods, is enough to restore your energy and health. The main thing is you learn to listen to your body and respond accordingly.

HOW TO EAT AFTER DETOXING?

Try to incorporate the main elements from this detox diet into your regular diet. Of course, you need not stick to the detox principles as rigidly as you have been. You are allowed a little more room for manoeuvre now that you have rid your body of excessive toxins.

● **Keep to the healthy eating principles at least 80% of the time.**

● **Re-introduce certain foods that you have missed to fill the remaining 20%. You may wish to include ordinary wheat bread or a wheat breakfast cereal in your diet. That should be fine provided you listen to your body. If you notice any symptoms, such as bloating or sluggishness, then cut back or eliminate.**

● **Avoid or minimise heavily processed foods for the first week or so. After this time, if you really want some chocolate, cake or whatever, have some. Just don't overdo it! You may find that you no longer crave the foods you used to or that they no longer make you feel satisfied.**

● It's best to reintroduce foods one at a time rather than eating them at once. That way, you will be able to work out which one(s) causes you unpleasant symptoms. Keep a food diary, if you can, noting down what you eat and how you feel.

● Vary your regular diet by incorporating more varieties of grains (rye, whole wheat, whole grain rice, corn, quinoa and millet), lean protein foods (fish, chicken, eggs, tofu, quorn and different beans and lentils), and dairy foods (skimmed milk, soya, rice, oat or almond milk, yoghurt or soya 'yoghurt'). If you suspect a food allergy or intolerance (e.g. dairy, gluten) you should consult a qualified nutritional practitioner for professional advice.

● Allow yourself occasional indulgences – whether it's chocolate, cheese, and wine – without feeling guilty. Most people who have completed a detox diet find that their craving is satisfied after eating or drinking only a very small amount. It is surprising how your taste buds change after eating super-healthily! Where before you may have eaten a whole chocolate bar (or more!), you may well find that a couple of squares of chocolate do the trick.

● Continue to listen to your body. If a certain food or drink doesn't feel 'right' or simply doesn't appeal, then don't have it. You should now be much more in tune with your body. Eat what your body really needs, savour your food and enjoy life!

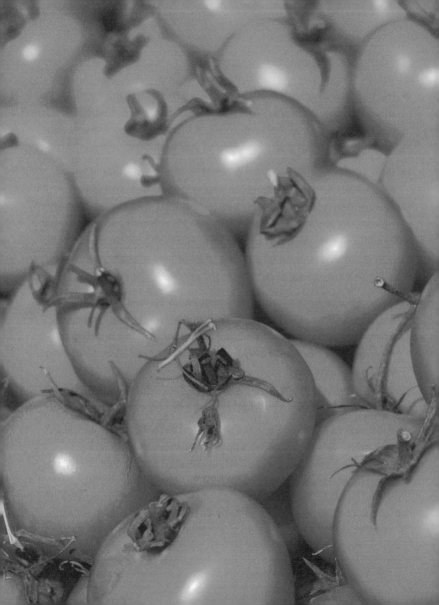

CHAPTER 9

THE DETOX PROGRAMME

You can follow my detox programme whenever you feel run-down and in need of an energy boost. I recommend you begin with a 7-day or 14-day detox – this is usually long enough to provide the energy boost your body needs.

I follow a 14-day detox twice a year, particularly before a holiday. I can lose quite a few inches of bloat and gain a much better complexion all over.

You can then try a longer detox if you're happy with the results from the short plan – provided you are feeling well and you include a wide variety of foods from the permitted list – for greater benefits or for more substantial weight loss. You can carry on with the programme for up to 28 days – it will do you the world of good and you'll never look back.

HOW TO EAT

Start each day with water, vegetable or fruit juice (opt for a juice with detoxing properties such as apple, carrot, cranberry, orange, grapefruit, pineapple or tomato), or herbal tea.

Eat three meals a day – breakfast, lunch and dinner. You can choose any of the meals in each of the three sections.

There are two sets of recipes. One set is marked with the symbol **D** for the strict detox and the other set marked **M** for maintenance. The **D** recipes in this book follow all the detox rules – no meat, fish, dairy, wheat, sugar or eggs. The **M** recipes are a little less strict and may include poultry, fish or low-fat dairy products. They are still well balanced but give you a little more room for manoeuvre.

Most of the recipes make 2 servings but you can adapt them by changing the quantities if you wish.

Space your meals through the day and if you can, try to make dinner the lightest meal of the day. The following recipes list lunch and dinner in the traditional way with a light lunch and a heavier dinner. Please try to swap these around as much as possible, having a heavier lunch and a lighter dinner as this will help your detoxing as much as possible. I have put them in the traditional order as I know how difficult this is for people at work who come home and want a rewarding dinner. If this is the case for you, don't worry but try to eat as early as you can and get some good rest.

Aim to drink at least 6 to 8 glasses of water or herbal tea (such as camomile, peppermint, dandelion and nettle) each day.

You can eat any fresh fruit for a between meal snack. Alternatively vegetable crudités with hummus or avocado dip; a small handful of unsalted nuts (plain or toasted); a small handful of (unsulphured) dried fruit; a small handful of seeds (plain or toasted); a glass of juice or a smoothie.

BREAKFAST

BREAKFAST SUGGESTIONS

1. Plate of fresh fruit, e.g. peaches, strawberries, kiwi fruit plus 1–2 tablespoons (15–30 ml) toasted almonds, hazelnuts or cashews, and 1 pot of bio-yoghurt or soya yoghurt

2. Sugar-free muesli with soya milk (or yoghurt) and raspberries

3. Slice of toast: rye bread or other non-wheat bread with olive oil spread and honey, plus ½ grapefruit

4. Plain soya or bio-yoghurt mixed with sliced banana and kiwi fruit

5. Porridge with raisins

6. Strawberry and banana smoothie plus a handful of nuts

GRANOLA WITH APPLE

This homemade granola is highly nutritious and contains much less sugar and oil than shop-bought versions. You can make larger quantities and store in an airtight container for up to 4 weeks.

D
Makes 2 servings

2 teaspoons (10 ml) clear honey
2 teaspoons (10 ml) sunflower oil
2 teaspoons (10 ml) lemon juice
1 teaspoon (5 ml) vanilla extract
½ tsp (2.5 ml) ground cinnamon
60 g (2 oz) oats

15 g (½ oz) sesame seeds
25 g (1 oz) hazelnuts, crushed
25 g (1 oz) mixed dried berries (or raisins)
1 apple, grated
natural bio-yoghurt

1. Heat the oven to 150 C/ 275 F/ Gas mark 1.

2. Combine the honey, oil, lemon juice, vanilla and cinnamon in a saucepan, then warm over a gentle heat until evenly mixed. Turn off the heat then mix in the oats, sesame seeds and hazelnuts.

3. Spread out on a non-stick baking tray and bake in the oven for 50–60 minutes, stirring occasionally until golden brown.

4. Cool and then mix in the dried berries. Store in an airtight container until ready to serve.

5. To serve, stir in the grated apple, spoon into bowls and top with a dollop of natural bio-yoghurt.

Health
Oats are rich in soluble fibre and provide slow-release energy as well as plenty of B vitamins and iron. Hazelnuts and sesame seeds provide protein, calcium, zinc and healthy monounsaturated oils. The apple provides extra fibre.

TOASTED PINEAPPLE AND PEACHES

Lightly toasted fresh fruit makes a welcome change from cereal at breakfast time.

D
Makes 2 servings

4 slices fresh pineapple, trimmed and core removed
2 peaches, skinned and halved
1 tablespoon (15 ml) sweet almond oil
25 g (1 oz) flaked toasted almonds

1. Preheat a hot grill. Arrange the fruit, cut side uppermost, on a foil-lined grill tray. Brush the cut sides with the almond oil. Grill for 2–3 minutes.

2. Arrange the toasted fruit on individual plates then sprinkle over the almond flakes. Serve immediately.

Health
Pineapple supplies vitamin C, fibre and potassium. It helps promote the detoxification process in the liver and also helps rid the body of excess fluid. The almonds supply extra protein and vitamin E.

MUESLI WITH FRESH FRUIT

D
Makes 2 servings

85 g (3 oz) mixture of oats, millet flakes and rye flakes
150 ml (¼ pint) soya, rice, almond or oat 'milk'
1 tablespoon (15 ml) each of toasted sunflower seeds and pumpkin seeds
25 g (1 oz) toasted flaked almonds
175–200 g (6–7 oz) fresh fruit, e.g. chopped mango, sliced bananas, strawberries,
   raspberries or blueberries

1. Place the cereal flakes in a bowl and pour the 'milk' over them. Leave to soak for at
least 2 hours, preferably overnight, in the fridge.

2. Stir in the seeds and almonds. Serve in individual bowls, topped with the fresh fruit.

> **Health**
> Oat and rye flakes are rich in soluble fibre, good for regulating blood sugar and
> insulin levels and reducing cholesterol levels. They also supply B vitamins, iron,
> magnesium and zinc. The seeds provide omega-3 and omega-6 fatty acids, to help
> balance hormone levels and promote overall good health. And the fresh fruit is rich in
> vitamin C, beta-carotene and fibre.

COMPOTE OF DRIED FRUIT

D
Makes 2 servings

150–175 g (5–6 oz) mixed dried fruits, e.g. figs, apricots, prunes, apples, mangos
300 ml (1/2 pint) boiling water
4 tablespoons (60 ml) soya or natural bio-yoghurt

1. Put the dried fruit in a large bowl. Cover with boiling water. Allow to cool, then cover and place in the fridge overnight. They should become plump and soft.

2. Drain the water. Spoon over the yoghurt.

Health
Dried fruit is super-rich in soluble fibre, which helps balance blood sugar levels, reduce cholesterol levels and promote healthy digestion. Figs are also rich in calcium and the dried apricots supply beta-carotene and iron. Prunes have one of the highest antioxidant scores of all fruits.

PORRIDGE WITH FRUIT

Starting the day with a bowl of porridge gives a great energy boost. Try adding sliced banana, blueberries, strawberries, clementine segments or any other fruit in season.

D
Makes 2 servings

85 g (3 oz) rolled porridge oats
125 ml (4 fl oz) skimmed, soya, rice, sesame or almond milk
125 ml (4 fl oz) water
2 tablespoons (30 ml) raisins, sultanas, dried apricots or dates
125 g (4 oz) fresh fruit (see above)
1 tablespoon (15 ml) honey

1. Mix the oats, milk and water in a saucepan. Bring to the boil and simmer for 4–5 minutes, stirring frequently.

2. Stir in the dried fruit. Spoon into bowls, drizzle over the honey and top with fresh fruit.

> **Health**
> Oats are rich in soluble fibre – excellent for improving digestion and lowering blood cholesterol – as well as iron, B vitamins, vitamin E and zinc. They provide slow-release energy to sustain your energy through the morning. The dried and fresh fruit provide extra fibre and vitamins.

OAT MUESLI WITH BERRIES

This recipe is prepared the evening before so you have an instant breakfast the next day. Soaking the oats overnight produces a softer and flavoursome muesli as they will have absorbed the liquid and flavours of the dried fruit. Alternatively use a ready-made muesli base then add your own nuts and fruit.

D
Makes 2 servings

85 g (3 oz) porridge oats (or other flaked cereal)
150 ml (¼ pint) skimmed, soya, rice, almond or oat 'milk'
2 tablespoons (30 ml) raisins (or other dried fruit)
2 tablespoons (30 ml) chopped brazils or walnuts
1 tablespoon (15 ml) ground linseeds (optional)
125 g (4 oz) blueberries, raspberries or strawberries

1. In a large bowl, mix together the oats (or other flakes), milk, dried fruit, nuts and ground linseeds. Cover and leave overnight in the fridge. Serve in individual bowls, topped with the fresh berries.

Health
Oats are rich in soluble fibre, which helps regulate blood sugar and insulin levels as well as reduce cholesterol levels. They also supply B vitamins, iron, magnesium and zinc. The nuts supply vitamin E, essential fatty acids and protein. Brazils are particularly good for selenium while walnuts and linseeds are excellent sources of omega-3 oils. The berries give you a great boost of vitamin C and cancer-protective phytonutrients.

BIO-YOGHURT WITH BANANA AND HONEY

Mix honey and fruit for a delicious and healthy start to the day. Adding live bio-yoghurt boosts the calcium and protein content.

M
Makes 2 servings

2 ripe bananas
300 g (10 oz) plain live bio-yoghurt or soya yoghurt
1–2 level tablespoons (15–30 ml) honey
2 tablespoons (30 ml) toasted flaked almonds (or walnuts, hazelnuts or pecans)

Slice the bananas into two bowls. Spoon half the yoghurt on top of each bowl. Drizzle with honey and scatter over the toasted nuts.

Health
Live bio-yoghurt contains health-boosting lactobacillus and bifida bacteria, which promote healthy digestion, help reduce bloating and boost your immune system. It's also a great source of protein and bone-strengthening calcium. Bananas supply fibre, potassium and vitamin B6 while the nuts add vitamin E and essential fatty acids.

LUNCH

LUNCH SUGGESTIONS

1. Carrot soup with 2 slices of rye bread, and a portion of fresh fruit

2. A small jacket potato with hummus and salad; and a portion of fresh fruit

3. Crudités (raw vegetable sticks) with avocado dip (guacamole), 1 slice of rye bread and fresh fruit

4. Leafy salad with cashew nuts, avocado and a little olive oil; a pot of bio-yoghurt or soya yoghurt

5. Open sandwich made with rye bread spread with hummus and topped with fresh tomatoes and red peppers, plus fresh fruit

6. Non-wheat pasta with chickpea and spinach salad

VEGETABLE STOCK

Use this stock for making soups, stews and casseroles in any recipes that call for stock. Alternatively, use 4 teaspoons (20 g) low-sodium vegetable bouillon powder dissolved in 1 litre of hot water.

Makes 600 ml (1 pint)

900 ml (1½ pints) water
2 onions, sliced
2 carrots, roughly sliced
2 celery sticks, halved
1 leek, halved
2 bay leaves
2 sprigs of thyme
2 sprigs of parsley
8 black peppercorns
pinch of sea salt to season

1. Put the water, vegetables, herbs and seasonings in a large saucepan.

2. Bring to the boil and simmer gently for at least 1 hour. Leave to cool and then strain.

CALDO VERDE

D
Makes 2 servings

1 tablespoon (15 ml) extra virgin olive oil
1 onion, chopped
1 garlic clove, crushed
225 g (8 oz) potatoes, peeled and diced
500 ml (16 fl oz) vegetable stock
225 g (8 oz) Savoy cabbage or spring greens, finely shredded
a little low-sodium salt and freshly ground black pepper, to taste

1. Heat the olive oil in a large heavy-based pan and cook the onion, garlic and potatoes over a moderate heat for about 5 minutes.

2. Add the stock and shredded cabbage, bring to the boil, and then simmer for 20 minutes until the vegetables are tender.

3. Remove half of the soup and liquidise using a hand blender or conventional blender. Return to the pan, stir well and reheat for a minute or two until piping hot. Season with low-sodium salt and black pepper.

Health
Savoy cabbage is rich in vitamin C and beta-carotene, which are both good immune-boosters. The outer green leaves of cabbage contain as much as 50 times the vitamins as inner white ones.

MEDITERRANEAN SUMMER VEGETABLE SOUP

D
Makes 2 servings

1 tablespoon (15 ml) extra virgin olive oil

1 onion, thinly sliced

1 garlic clove, finely chopped

half a red and half a green pepper, deseeded and sliced

1 courgette, trimmed and sliced

225 g (8 oz) tomatoes, skinned and quartered

half an aubergine, diced

500 ml (16 fl oz) vegetable stock or water

a little low-sodium salt, to taste

2 teaspoons (10 ml) pesto

1. Heat the olive oil in a large saucepan. Add the onion and garlic and sauté over a moderate heat for about 5 minutes until it is translucent.

2. Add the prepared vegetables, stock or water, then bring to the boil. Simmer for about 25–30 minutes or until the vegetables are tender.

3. Allow the soup to cool slightly for a couple of minutes. Liquidise the soup using a hand blender or conventional blender. Season to taste with low-sodium salt.

4. Serve in individual bowls, adding a teaspoon of pesto to each bowl immediately before serving.

Health
This dish is rich in vitamin C (from the tomatoes and peppers), beta-carotene and lycopene (both from the tomatoes), a powerful antioxidant that helps to protect against heart disease and several cancers. It is also an excellent source of potassium, good for regulating fluid balance and controlling blood pressure.

EASY CARROT SOUP

One of the easiest vegetable soups to make and packed with vital nutrients, this is a firm winter favourite.

D
Makes 2 servings

1 onion, finely chopped
1 garlic clove, crushed
4 carrots, sliced
1 medium potato, peeled and chopped
  500 ml (16 fl oz) vegetable stock
freshly ground black pepper
1 tablespoon (15 ml) omega-3 rich oil or olive oil
1 tablespoon (15 ml) fresh parsley, finely chopped

1. Place the onion, garlic, carrots and potatoes in a large saucepan. Add the stock and bring to the boil, then reduce the heat and simmer for 15 minutes until the vegetables are tender.

2. Allow the soup to cool slightly for a couple of minutes. Season with freshly ground black pepper and add the oil.

3. Liquidise the soup using a hand blender or conventional blender, then stir in the fresh parsley.

Health
This soup is an excellent source of beta-carotene, a powerful antioxidant that helps combat free radicals that cause cancer. It is also good for strengthening the skin and boosting its natural defences against the damaging effects of ultraviolet light.

SPICY LENTIL SOUP

This soup is hearty and filling. You can add extra vegetables, such as carrots and mushrooms, to boost the nutritional and fibre value.

D
Makes 2 servings

1–2 teaspoons (5–10 ml) curry paste
1 onion, chopped
1 garlic clove, crushed
2 cm piece root ginger, peeled and finely chopped
125 g (4 oz) red lentils
500 ml (16 fl oz) vegetable stock
grated zest and juice of 1 lime
a little low-sodium salt and freshly ground black pepper
chopped fresh mint to garnish

1. Place the curry paste, onion, garlic and ginger in a large pan and cook gently for 3 minutes.

2. Add the lentils and vegetable stock and bring to the boil. Reduce the heat and simmer for 20 minutes. Add the lime zest and juice, bring back to the boil and simmer for a further 10 minutes until the lentils are soft. Season to taste with low-sodium salt and pepper.

3. Ladle into bowls and garnish with the mint.

> **Health**
> Lentils are low in fat and high in protein as well as an excellent source of complex carbohydrates and fibre. They also supply iron, B vitamins, zinc and selenium, which make them powerful nutrient powerhouses.

ITALIAN BEAN SOUP

This variation of minestrone soup is fantastically satisfying. You can substitute borlotti beans if you wish.

D
Makes 2 servings

1 garlic clove, crushed
1 small onion, finely chopped
½ leek, finely chopped
1 carrot, peeled and chopped
400 g (14 oz) can cannelloni beans, rinsed and drained
500 ml (16 fl oz) vegetable stock
1 bay leaf

½ teaspoon (2.5 ml) dried sage, crushed
2 tablespoons (30 ml) chopped fresh flat-leaf parsley, plus extra to garnish
freshly ground black pepper
1 tablespoon (15 ml) omega 3-rich oil or extra virgin olive oil

1. Place the garlic, vegetables, beans, vegetable stock, bay leaf and sage in a large saucepan. Bring to the boil, lower the heat, cover and simmer for about 20 minutes until the vegetables are tender.

2. Remove from the heat and remove the bay leaf. Stir in the fresh parsley. Season with freshly ground black pepper and ladle into warmed bowls. Scatter over the extra parsley and drizzle with the oil before serving.

Health
This soup provides plenty of fibre (from the vegetables and the beans), important for efficient digestive function and colon health. The type of fibre provided by beans also helps lower blood cholesterol levels and protects against heart disease. They also supply good amounts of protein, complex carbohydrate, B vitamins and zinc.

AVOCADO AND WALNUT SALAD

Avocados are one of my favourite salad ingredients not only because they taste divine, but also because they keep you feeling satisfied for a long time.

D
Makes 2 servings

1 avocado, peeled, stoned and halved
1 tablespoon (15 ml) lemon juice
2–3 handfuls salad leaves, e.g. rocket, watercress, lettuce
60 g (2 oz) walnut halves
Dressing
1 tablespoon (15 ml) walnut oil
1 tablespoon (15 ml) olive oil
2 teaspoons (10 ml) cider vinegar
1 teaspoon (5 ml) lemon juice

1. Cut avocados into slices and turn gently in lemon juice to stop them discolouring.

2. Place the mixed salad leaves in the serving dish. Arrange the avocado slices on top and sprinkle over the walnuts.

3. Shake the dressing ingredients together in a screw-top glass jar. Drizzle over the salad.

> **Health**
> Avocados are excellent for your skin, helping to keep it smooth and prevent wrinkles. They are full of heart-healthy monounsaturated oils and vitamin E. The walnut oil in the dressing supplies extra omega-3 oils, which are also great for supple skin as well as preventing strokes and heart attacks.

CHAR-GRILLED VEGETABLE SALAD WITH ROCKET AND PINE NUTS

This salad can be varied infinitely according to which vegetables you have handy.

D
Makes 2 servings

1 courgette, sliced lengthways
½ aubergine, cut into thin slices
1 red pepper, deseeded and cut into wide strips
2 plum tomatoes
1 tablespoon (15 ml) extra virgin olive oil
1 bag (50 g) rocket
2 tablespoons (30 ml) pine nuts

1 tablespoon (15 ml) basil leaves, torn
Dressing
1 tablespoon (15 ml) extra virgin olive oil
1 teaspoon (5 ml) lemon juice
½ teaspoon (2.5 ml) wholegrain mustard
freshly ground black pepper

1. Preheat the grill.

2. Place the vegetables on a baking tray. Drizzle over the olive oil, and turn the vegetables gently so they are lightly coated in the oil. Grill the vegetables for around 2 minutes each side (or until slightly browned), turning once to cook on both sides. Allow to cool.

3. Place the rocket in a large salad bowl. Add the grilled vegetables and pine nuts.

4. To make the dressing, place the olive oil, lemon juice, mustard and black pepper in a screw-top glass jar and shake well until mixed. Pour the dressing over the salad, toss well and scatter over the torn basil leaves.

Health
This fibre-rich salad provides lots of vitamin C and beta-carotene, both powerful antioxidants that are protective against heart disease and many cancers.

RICE AND BROAD BEAN SALAD WITH BALSAMIC DRESSING

Here's a salad you can throw together from your store cupboard ingredients.

D
Makes 2 servings

125 g (4 oz) wholegrain (brown) rice
300 g (10 oz) can broad beans, rinsed and drained (or use cooked frozen beans)
125 g (4 oz) canned sweetcorn, rinsed and drained
125 g (4 oz) baby plum tomatoes, halved
1 red pepper, cut into strips
1 tablespoon (15 ml) capers (optional)
2 tablespoons (30 ml) extra virgin olive oil
1 tablespoon (15 ml) balsamic vinegar
½ teaspoon (2.5 ml) wholegrain mustard

1. Bring a large pan of water to the boil. Stir in the rice. Cover and simmer for the time recommended on the packet. Drain. Alternatively, cook the rice in twice its own volume of water until the water has been absorbed.

2. Place the cooled rice in a large bowl with the broad beans and sweetcorn.

3. Add the plum tomatoes and red pepper to the rice mixture along with the capers, if using, and mix together.

4. To make the dressing, put the oil, vinegar and mustard in a screw-top glass jar and shake well. Drizzle over the salad, toss well and serve.

> **Health**
> Broad beans are rich in soluble fibre, which helps control blood cholesterol levels and is also responsible for their low GI.

CARROT AND ALMOND SALAD

D
Makes 2 servings

2 large carrots
half an orange
half a lemon or lime
25 g (1 oz) raisins
2 tablespoons (30 ml) extra virgin olive oil
1 tablespoon (15 ml) toasted flaked almonds

1. Scrub or peel the carrots and grate them coarsely.

2. Scrub the orange and lemon or lime, then finely grate the rind and add it to the carrots. Toss through the carrots then stir in the raisins.

3. Squeeze the orange and lemon or lime and mix the juice with the extra virgin olive oil in a screw-top glass jar.

4. Pour the dressing over the carrot salad. Scatter over the toasted flaked almonds and serve.

Health
Carrots are one of the best detoxifying foods, helping to cleanse the body. And it's true that they can help you to see in the dark as they are packed with beta-carotene, needed for vision in dim light. Just one medium carrot gives you your daily requirement for beta-carotene.

CHICKPEA AND RED PEPPER SALAD WITH WALNUTS

D
Makes 2 servings

200 g (7 oz) tinned chickpeas, drained and rinsed
half a red onion, thinly sliced
half red pepper, deseeded and sliced
6 black olives, pitted
1 packet (100 g) of ready-washed watercress
40 g (½ oz) walnuts, lightly toasted
Dressing
2 tablespoons (30 ml) extra virgin olive oil
1 tablespoon (15 ml) balsamic vinegar
1 small garlic clove, crushed
half a teaspoon (2.5 ml) Dijon mustard

1. In a large bowl, mix together the chickpeas, onion, pepper and olives.

2. Place the dressing ingredients in a screw-top glass jar and shake until combined. Add half of the dressing to the chickpea salad and mix until well combined.

3. Toss the watercress with the remaining dressing. Transfer to a serving plate. Top with the chickpea salad and sprinkle with the toasted walnuts.

Health
Chickpeas are an excellent source of fibre, protein and iron. Watercress is also rich in iron as well as vitamin C, beta-carotene and folate.

WHOLEGRAIN RICE WITH ROASTED PEPPERS, TOMATOES AND MINT

D
Makes 2 servings

half a small red pepper, deseeded and cut into wide strips
half a small yellow pepper, deseeded and cut into wide strips
125 g (4 oz) cherry tomatoes, halved
1 tablespoon (15 ml) extra virgin olive oil
125 g (4 oz) brown (wholegrain) rice
150 ml (4 fl oz) hot vegetable stock or water
200 g (7 oz) tin red kidney beans, drained and rinsed
a small handful of fresh mint, chopped
a little low-sodium salt and freshly ground black pepper

1. Preheat the oven to 200 C/ 400 F/ Gas mark 6.

2. Place the peppers in a large roasting tin with the cherry tomatoes, drizzle over the olive oil and toss lightly so that the vegetables are well coated in the oil. Roast in the oven for about 30 minutes until the peppers are slightly charred on the outside and tender in the middle. Allow to cool then roughly chop the peppers.

3. Add the rice to a large pan of water and bring to the boil. Reduce the heat and simmer for 30–35 minutes until the grains are tender. Drain and fluff the rice.

4. Add the roast peppers, tomatoes, beans and mint. Season to taste with low-sodium salt and black pepper. Serve.

Health
The red kidney beans are rich in protein, fibre, zinc and iron.

RATATOUILLE

D
Makes 4 servings

1 tablespoon (15 ml) extra virgin olive oil
1 onion, peeled and chopped
half each of red, yellow and green peppers, deseeded and sliced
1 clove of garlic, crushed
1 large courgette, sliced
half aubergine, diced
400 g (14 oz) tomatoes, skinned and chopped (or use 400 g/ 14 oz can tomatoes)
sea salt and freshly ground black pepper
1 tablespoon (15 ml) chopped fresh parsley

1. Heat the oil in a large saucepan. Add the onions and peppers and cook gently for 5 minutes.

2. Add the garlic, courgette, aubergine and tomatoes. Stir, then cover and cook over a low heat for 20–25 minutes until all the vegetables are tender.

3. Season to taste with salt and freshly ground black pepper and sprinkle with the chopped parsley. Serve hot or cold.

Health
This delicious Provencal vegetable dish is packed with powerful antioxidants, including vitamin C (in the peppers), nasuin (in the aubergines) and quercetin (in the onions). Together they make a potent anti-cancer cocktail of nutrients.

GREEK SALAD WITH FENNEL AND MINT

M
Makes 2 servings

half a romaine lettuce
1 small bulb of fennel
20 cm (8 in) length cucumber
1–2 large tomatoes
half a green, red or orange pepper
1 small red onion
handful of fresh mint, roughly torn
85 g (3 oz) feta cheese
60 g (2 oz) black kalamata olives

Dressing
2 tablespoons (30 ml) extra virgin olive
   oil
juice of half a lemon
a small bunch of flat-leaf parsley,
   chopped
a little low-sodium salt and freshly
   ground black pepper, to taste

1. Cut the lettuce into wide ribbons. Halve, then thinly slice the fennel, discarding the tough inner 'core'. Cut the cucumber lengthways in half then half again, and then slice thickly. Cut the tomatoes into quarters. Remove the seeds from the pepper and slice it thinly. Slice the onion thinly.

2. Put the prepared vegetables into a large bowl. Add the mint leaves, feta and olives.

3. Whisk the dressing ingredients together in a small bowl. Pour the dressing over the salad and toss well.

Health
This salad is rich in potassium and vitamin C. The dark green leaves of the romaine lettuce provide beta-carotene and iron and the peppers and tomatoes are super-rich in vitamin C. Feta cheese is made from sheep or goat's milk and contains 20% fat, which is considerably lower than other hard cheeses (around 30%).

SEA BASS WITH SPRING VEGETABLES

M
Makes 2 servings

2 x 250 g (9 oz) sea bass fillets
1 tablespoon (15 ml) extra virgin olive oil
60 g (2 oz) fine green beans, trimmed and cut into 5 cm (2 inch) lengths
60 g (2 oz) sugar-snap peas, trimmed
60 g (2 oz) asparagus, trimmed and cut into 5 cm (2 inch) lengths
85 g (3 oz) fresh or frozen broad beans
200 g (7 oz) tinned flageolet beans, drained and rinsed

1. Heat the oven to 180 C/ 350 F/ Gas mark 4.

2. Pan fry each sea bass fillet in the olive oil for a minute each side to seal, then transfer on to a baking tray and finish cooking in the oven for 8–10 minutes.

3. Steam or boil the green beans, sugar-snap peas, asparagus and broad beans for 4 minutes until they are tender-crisp. Add the flageolet beans one minute before the end of the cooking time so they heat through.

4. Place the sea bass in the centre of each plate then scatter the vegetables around. Serve immediately.

> **Health**
> The sea bass is rich in protein and B vitamins, while the vegetables provide plenty of fibre, potassium and protective antioxidants.

GRILLED RED PEPPERS WITH RICOTTA AND BASIL

D
Makes 2 servings

2 red large peppers
1 tablespoon (15 ml) extra virgin olive oil
85 g (3 oz) ricotta cheese
a little low-sodium salt and freshly ground black pepper
a small handful of fresh basil leaves, chopped
Tomato sauce
1 tbsp (15 ml) extra virgin olive oil
1 onion, chopped
1 garlic cloves, crushed
225 g (8 oz) ripe tomatoes, skinned, deseeded and chopped, or 400 g (14 oz)
    tinned chopped tomatoes
a little low-sodium salt and freshly ground black pepper

1. Preheat the grill.

2. Brush the peppers with a little of the olive oil, place them in a shallow tin, then place under the grill, turning frequently, until blistered and blackened all over. Put in a bowl, cover with cling film and leave to cool. Carefully remove the skin. Cut each pepper into quarters lengthways removing the seeds.

3. Heat the oven to 200 C/ 400 F/ gas mark 6.

4. Season the ricotta with low-sodium salt and pepper and mix in the basil. Take a heaped teaspoon of the mixture and place at the narrow end of each pepper. Roll up and place in an ovenproof dish.

5. Brush each pepper with olive oil and place the dish in the oven for 10 minutes.

6. Meanwhile, make the tomato sauce. Heat the olive oil in a heavy-based frying pan. Add the onion and garlic and cook over a low heat for 5 minutes until soft and transparent. Add the chopped tomatoes. Bring to the boil, reduce the heat and simmer for 10 minutes, stirring occasionally. Season with a little salt and black pepper.

7. Serve with the grilled peppers.

Health
Red peppers are super-rich in vitamin C, beta-cryptoxanthin and beta-carotene, all powerful antioxidants that help protect the body from heart disease and cancer. Ricotta cheese is relatively low in fat (11%) and provides protein and calcium.

DINNER

DINNER SUGGESTIONS

1. Vegetable and cashew nut stir fry with noodles, plus fresh fruit salad

2. Tofu and vegetable kebabs with cous cous, plus baked bananas

3. Lentil and rocket salad, plus a bowl of strawberries

4. Wholegrain rice pilaf with green beans and nuts

5. A jacket potato, stir fried vegetables and toasted seeds

6. Non-wheat pasta with vegetables and red kidney beans

SPICED QUINOA PILAFF

This is one of my favourite ways of serving quinoa. It's very easy to make as everything is cooked in one pan. You can add other vegetables such as peas and green beans, and a handful of toasted cashews or walnuts.

D

Makes 2 servings

1 tablespoon (15 ml) extra virgin olive oil
1 small onion, chopped
1 garlic clove, crushed
1 teaspoon (5 ml) cumin seeds
½ teaspoon (2.5 ml) turmeric
1 red pepper, deseeded and chopped

125 g (4 oz) quinoa
600 ml (1 pint) vegetable stock
a little low-sodium salt and freshly ground black pepper
2 tablespoons (30 ml) sultanas
handful of fresh coriander leaves, roughly chopped

1. Heat the oil in a large saucepan and sauté the onion over a gentle heat for 5 minutes.

2. Add the garlic, cumin seeds, turmeric and pepper and continue cooking for 3 minutes. Add the quinoa and vegetable stock, stir well, then bring to the boil. Reduce the heat and simmer for about 20 minutes until the liquid has been absorbed and the grains are tender.

3. Season with low sodium salt and black pepper. Stir in the sultanas and coriander.

4. Serve with lightly steamed vegetables and grilled fish, chicken or tofu.

> **Health**
> Quinoa has a low GI so will make you feel satisfied for longer, prevent hunger and keep your blood sugar levels steady. It provides a good source of protein, magnesium, zinc, fibre and vitamin E. The pepper provides plenty of vitamin C, which is good for strengthening collagen and the walls of your small blood vessels.

SPAGHETTI WITH FRESH TOMATOES AND BASIL

Make this simple dish in the summer when fresh tomatoes are plentiful and full of flavour.
Serve with a leafy salad.

D

Makes 2 servings

4 medium vine-ripened tomatoes
175 g (6 oz) non-wheat spaghetti
small handful fresh basil leaves
2 tablespoons (30 ml) extra virgin olive oil
a little low sodium salt and freshly ground black pepper
25 g (1 oz) pine nuts, lightly toasted

1. To skin the tomatoes, place them in a bowl and pour over boiling water, leave for
one minute, and then drain off the water. Pierce the skin with a sharp knife and the skin
should slide off quite easily. Chop the tomatoes roughly.

2. Cook the pasta in boiling water according to the packet instructions. Drain and return
to the saucepan. Add the chopped tomatoes, roughly torn basil leaves, olive oil and
seasoning. Stir well to mix over a gentle heat for a minute to heat through. Divide between
two bowls and scatter over the pine nuts.

Health
Fresh tomatoes are rich in immune-boosting vitamin C – this recipe supplies 27
mg vitamin C, approximately 70% of your daily needs. Vitamin C helps strengthen
collagen and thus improve the appearance of cellulite. They also provide good
amounts of vitamin E and potassium. Fresh basil supplies extra beta-carotene
and iron.

LENTIL AND VEGETABLE DAHL WITH CASHEW NUTS

D
Makes 2 servings

1 tablespoon (15 ml) rapeseed oil
1 onion, chopped
1 garlic clove, crushed
½ teaspoon (2.5 ml) ground cumin
1 teaspoon (5 ml) ground coriander
½ teaspoon (2.5 ml) turmeric
85 g (3 oz) red lentils
350 ml (12 fl oz) vegetable stock

1–2 carrots, diced
1 courgette, sliced
60 g (2 oz) frozen peas
125 g (4 oz) cashew nuts, toasted
1 tablespoon (15 ml) lemon juice
a little low-sodium salt
a small handful of fresh coriander,
    finely chopped

1. Heat the oil in a heavy-based pan and sauté the onion for 5 minutes. Add the garlic and spices and continue cooking for one minute while stirring continuously.

2. Add the lentils, stock, carrots and courgette. Bring to the boil. Cover and simmer for about 20 minutes, adding the peas 5 minutes before the end of the cooking time.

3. Stir in the cashew nuts then season with the lemon juice and low-sodium salt. Finally, stir in the fresh coriander.

Health
Red lentils are rich in protein, complex carbohydrates and soluble fibre. They provide slow-release energy and help balance blood sugar levels. Red lentils are also rich in iron, zinc and B vitamins. Cashews supply further protein and zinc.

CHICK PEAS WITH SPINACH AND POTATO

D
Makes 2 servings

1 tablespoon (15 ml) extra virgin olive oil
1 onion, chopped
1 garlic clove, crushed
1 red pepper, deseeded and chopped
2 medium potatoes, peeled and cut into 2 cm (1 in) chunks

400 g (14 oz) tinned chopped tomatoes
125 ml (4 fl oz) vegetable stock
400 g (14 oz) tinned chick peas, drained and rinsed
85 g (3 oz) fresh spinach, washed and trimmed

1. Heat the oil in a heavy-based pan, add the onion, garlic and red pepper, and cook over a moderate heat for 5 minutes.

2. Add the potatoes, tinned tomatoes, vegetable stock and chickpeas, stir then bring to the boil. Lower the heat and simmer for 20 minutes, stirring occasionally.

3. Stir in the spinach, cover and continue cooking for a few minutes until the spinach is wilted.

4. Serve in individual bowls.

Health
Chickpeas are an excellent source of fibre, protein and iron. They also contain fructo-oligosaccharides, a type of fibre that maintains healthy gut flora and increases the friendly bacteria of the gut – especially useful if your gut bacteria get upset by travel or stress.

NEST OF STIR-FRIED VEGETABLES ON RICE

D
Makes 2 servings

1 tablespoon (15 ml) olive oil
1 teaspoon (5 ml) sesame oil
1 small onion, sliced
1 teaspoon (5 ml) grated fresh ginger
1 garlic clove, crushed
½ red pepper, sliced

1 carrot, cut into thin batons
1 courgette, sliced
85 g (3 oz) button mushrooms
2 tablespoons (30 ml) pine nuts
125 g (4 oz) brown or wild rice

1. Heat the oils in a non-stick wok or large frying pan. Add the onion, ginger and garlic and stir-fry for 2 minutes.

2. Add the pepper and carrot and stir-fry for a further 2–3 minutes.

3. Add the remaining vegetables and continue stir-frying for a further 2 minutes. Stir in the pine nuts.

4. Wash the rice. Add to a large pan of water and bring to the boil. Reduce the heat and simmer for 30–35 minutes until the grains are tender. Drain and fluff the rice. Arrange a circular nest of rice on two plates. Fill each rice nest with the stir-fried vegetables and serve immediately.

Health
Stir-frying helps preserve the vitamins in the vegetables because they are cooked only briefly at a high temperature and no vitamins are lost in cooking liquid. This recipe is a good source of vitamin C, fibre and vitamin E.

TOFU AND MUSHROOM KEBABS

D
Makes 2 servings

Marinade
2 tablespoons (30 ml) olive oil
1 tablespoon (15 ml) low sodium soy
   sauce
½ teaspoon (2.5 ml) grated fresh root
   ginger
1 teaspoon (5 ml) clear honey
1 garlic clove, crushed

1–2 tablespoons (15–30 ml) water
125 g (4 oz) firm tofu (plain or
   smoked), cut into chunks
1 red or yellow pepper, de-seeded and
   cut into 2.5 cm (1 inch) pieces
½ aubergine, cut into bite-sized pieces
16 button mushrooms

1. To make the marinade, mix together the olive oil, soy sauce, ginger, honey, garlic and water.

2. Place the tofu, peppers, aubergine and mushrooms in a shallow dish, pour over the marinade, turn gently, making sure they are thoroughly coated. Leave covered for about 30 minutes (or longer), turning occasionally.

3. Preheat the grill and line the grill rack with foil.

4. Thread the tofu and vegetables onto 4 wooden skewers. Brush with the remaining marinade and place under the hot grill for about 10 minutes, turning frequently and brushing with marinade, until slightly browned.

5. Serve with cooked wholegrain rice and a green salad.

Health
Marinating vegetables in olive oil before grilling is healthy because the oil is mostly the healthy monounsaturated kind, which features heavily in the Mediterranean diet.

RISOTTO WITH ASPARAGUS AND PEAS

D
Makes 2 servings

1 tablespoon (15 ml) extra virgin olive oil
2 shallots, chopped (or 1 onion)
150 g (5 oz) Arborio (risotto) rice
500 ml (16 fl oz) hot vegetable stock
125 g (4 oz) asparagus, cut into 4 cm (1½ inch) lengths

60 g (2 oz) fresh or frozen peas
finely grated zest of one lemon
handful of fresh basil leaves, torn
a little low sodium salt and black pepper

1. Heat the olive oil in a large pan. Add the shallots and cook for 2 minutes until translucent.

2. Add the rice and stir with a wooden spoon until the grains are coated with the oil.

3. Stir in the hot vegetable stock one ladle at a time and simmer for about 10 minutes.

4. Add the asparagus, peas and lemon zest. Continue cooking for a further 10 minutes until all the liquid has been absorbed and the rice is tender but firm in the centre.

5. Stir in the basil leaves and season to taste. Serve immediately.

Health
Asparagus is a good source of folic acid and vitamin E. It also contains fructo-oligosaccharides, a type of fibre that helps maintain a healthy gut flora and lower cholesterol levels.

BEAN PROVENCAL WITH BLACK OLIVES

D

Makes 2 servings

1 tablespoon (15 ml) extra virgin olive oil
1 onion, sliced
half a red pepper, deseeded and sliced
half a green pepper, deseeded and sliced
1 garlic clove, crushed
1 courgette, trimmed and sliced
200 g (7 oz) tinned chopped tomatoes
200 g (7 oz) tinned cannellini beans or butter beans
1 tablespoon (15 ml) tomato paste
1 teaspoon (5 ml) dried oregano or basil
30 g (1 oz) black olives
a little low-sodium salt and freshly ground black pepper
a small handful of fresh parsley or basil leaves, chopped

1. Heat the olive oil in a heavy-based pan and sauté the onions and peppers over a moderate heat until soft. Add the garlic and courgette and continue cooking for a further 5 minutes, stirring occasionally.

2. Add the tomatoes, beans, tomato paste and dried herbs. Cover and simmer for 15–20 minutes, adding the olives 5 minutes before the end of the cooking time. Season with the low-sodium salt and black pepper. Serve sprinkled with the parsley or basil leaves.

Health
Cannellini beans are rich in protein, complex carbohydrate and soluble fibre, which help balance blood sugar and insulin levels. The peppers are super-rich in vitamin C, a powerful antioxidant that helps prevent cancer and heart disease. Olives supply plenty of heart-healthy monounsaturated fats and vitamin E.

VEGETABLE CURRY WITH BLACK EYE BEANS AND ALMONDS

D
Makes 2 servings

1 carrot, sliced
1 medium potato, peeled and cubed
½ butternut squash, peeled and cut
   into cubes
125 g (4 oz) broccoli florets
60 g (2 oz) frozen peas
2 tablespoons (30 ml) olive oil
1 onion, sliced
½ teaspoon (2.5 ml) of each: cumin,
   coriander and turmeric
1 garlic clove, crushed
1 teaspoon (5 ml) grated fresh ginger

200 g (7 oz) tinned chopped tomatoes
1 tablespoon (15 ml) desiccated
   coconut
200 ml (7 fl oz) plain yoghurt
25 g (1 oz) ground almonds
225 g (8 oz) tinned black eye beans,
   rinsed and drained
small handful fresh coriander leaves,
   chopped
a little low sodium salt and freshly
   ground black pepper

1. Boil or steam the carrot, potato, butternut squash and broccoli for 5 minutes. Add the peas and cook for a further 3 minutes. Drain the vegetables and put aside.

2. Heat the oil in a large pan and add the onion. Cook gently for 5 minutes until softened. Add the spices, garlic and ginger and cook for a further minute then add the tomatoes. Bring to the boil and cook for 2–3 minutes.

3. In a separate bowl, mix together the coconut, yoghurt and almonds.

4. Add the cooked vegetables and black eye beans to the tomato mixture and simmer for a few minutes. Finally, stir in the yoghurt mixture. Turn off the heat, taking care not to boil otherwise the yoghurt may curdle. Stir in the coriander and season with low sodium salt and freshly ground black pepper. Serve with brown rice.

PASTA SPIRALS WITH GRILLED VEGETABLES

D
Makes 2 servings

½ red pepper, cut into wide strips
½ yellow pepper, cut into wide strips
1 small courgette, thinly sliced lengthways
1 small red onion, thinly sliced
4 tomatoes, halved
extra virgin olive oil, for brushing
175 g (6 oz) non-wheat pasta spirals
handful of fresh basil leaves

1. Preheat the grill to high. Arrange the pepper strips, courgette, onion and tomato halves in a single layer on a grill pan. Brush with a little olive oil and grill for 2 minutes on each side.

2. Meanwhile, cook the pasta in boiling water according to the packet instructions. Drain then combine with the cooked vegetable mixture.

3. Scatter over the basil leaves.

> **Health**
> Red and yellow peppers are super-rich in vitamin C and beta-carotene, both powerful antioxidants with anti-cancer effects. Courgettes are rich in potassium, which helps to balance fluid levels in the body.

RICE NOODLES WITH VEGETABLES IN SPICED COCONUT MILK

D
Makes 2 servings

85 g (3 oz) rice noodles
1 tablespoon (5 ml) olive oil
1 small onion, chopped
1 garlic clove, finely chopped
½ teaspoon (2.5 ml) grated fresh
  ginger
1 teaspoon (5 ml) ground coriander

pinch of ground turmeric
200 ml (7 fl oz) coconut milk
125 ml (4 fl oz) vegetable stock
85 g (3 oz) green beans
125 g (4 oz) green cabbage, shredded
small handful of fresh coriander,
  chopped

1. Cook the noodles according to the instructions on the packet. Drain.

2. Heat the oil in a wok or large saucepan. Add the onion, garlic, ginger, ground coriander and turmeric and stir-fry for a few minutes. Add the coconut milk and stock and bring to the boil. Reduce the heat and stir in the green beans, cabbage and cooked noodles. Cover and simmer for 5 minutes.

3. Stir in the coriander and serve in individual bowls.

> **Health**
> Coconut milk contains high levels of potassium, good for ridding the body of excess fluid, and is also very low in fat. This dish provides fibre and vitamin C.

DAHL WITH SWEET POTATOES AND COCONUT

D
Makes 2 servings

1 onion, chopped
85 g (3o z) red lentils
200 ml (7 fl oz) coconut milk
225 ml (8 fl oz) water
1 sweet potato (weighing approx 250 g/ 9 oz)
1–2 garlic cloves, crushed
½ teaspoon (2.5 ml) fresh grated ginger
½ teaspoon (2.5 ml) ground cumin
1 teaspoon (5 ml) ground coriander
¼ teaspoon (1.25 ml) turmeric
a little low sodium salt and freshly ground black pepper
handful of fresh coriander or parsley, finely chopped

1. Put the onion, lentils, coconut milk, water, sweet potato and garlic in a large saucepan. Bring to the boil, then lower the heat and simmer gently for 20 minutes until the lentils and sweet potatoes are tender. The dhal will be quite thick, like porridge.

2. Stir in the ginger, spices, low sodium salt and pepper and cook for a few more minutes. Stir in the coriander and serve with steamed green cabbage or broccoli.

> **Health**
> Red lentils are a good source of protein, complex carbohydrate, fibre, iron and B vitamins. The sweet potato provides good amounts of beta-carotene, useful for helping protect against cancer and heart disease.

FISH STEW WITH FENNEL AND TOMATOES

M
Makes 2 servings

1 tablespoon (15 ml) extra virgin olive oil
1 fennel bulb, finely sliced
1 garlic clove, crushed
250 ml (8 fl oz) fish or vegetable stock
400 g (14 oz) tinned chopped tomatoes
125 g (4 oz) cherry tomatoes, halved
a little low-sodium salt and freshly ground black pepper
25 g (8 oz) monkfish fillet, cut into 4 cm (2 in) chunks
1 tablespoon (15 ml) chopped chives

1. Heat the olive oil in a large pan, add the fennel and cook over a moderate heat for 5 minutes. Add the garlic and cook for a further minute.

2. Stir in the stock and tinned tomatoes, bring to the boil and simmer gently for 5 minutes.

3. Add the cherry tomatoes and cook for a further 5 minutes. Season with low-sodium salt and freshly ground pepper.

4. Add the monkfish, cover and cook for approximately 5 minutes or until the fish is cooked. Serve the stew in individual bowls and garnish with the chopped chives.

Health
This dish is rich in protein and B vitamins (from the fish). Fennel provides folate and potassium and the tomatoes are rich in vitamin C and lycopene, a powerful antioxidant nutrient that helps fight cancer.

BREAST OF CHICKEN WITH BUTTERNUT SQUASH MASH

M
Makes 2 servings

2 medium potatoes
2 chicken breasts on the bone
a little extra virgin olive oil
half a butternut squash
3 tablespoons (45 ml) skimmed milk
a little low-sodium salt and freshly ground black pepper
a small handful of fresh flat-leaf parsley, chopped

1. Heat the oven to 190 C/ 375 F/ Gas mark 5.

2. Scrub and prick the potatoes and cook in the oven for 45–60 minutes, depending on the size of the potatoes.

3. Meanwhile, place the chicken breasts in a roasting tin, drizzle over a little olive oil, turn the chicken so that they are well coated with oil.

4. Peel the butternut squash and cut the flesh into large chunks. Place in a separate baking tin, drizzle over a little oil and toss until well coated.

5. Cook the chicken and the squash in the oven for 20–30 minutes, depending on the size of the chicken breasts. The squash should be soft but not mushy.

6. Halve the potatoes and scoop out the flesh into a bowl. Add the cooked squash and milk, season with the salt and pepper and mash until smooth. Adjust the consistency with a little extra milk if you wish.

7. Divide the mash between four plates and place a chicken breast on top. Scatter over the chopped flat-leaf parsley and serve immediately.

Health
Butternut squash is super-rich in beta-carotene, which has powerful antioxidant properties, helping protect against heart disease and cancer. The potatoes provide complex carbohydrates, fibre and vitamin C. Chicken is rich in protein and B vitamins.

OAT-CRUSTED SALMON WITH SESAME SEEDS

The lightly toasted oat crust makes the fish lovely and crispy on the outside while adding extra flavour and nutrients. Serve this dish with steamed new potatoes and a salad of watercress and spinach.

M
Makes 2 servings

300 g (10 oz) salmon fillet, skinned
2 tablespoons (30 ml) porridge oats
1 tablespoon (15 ml) sesame seeds
a little low sodium salt and freshly ground black pepper
lemon wedges to serve

1. Cut the salmon in half.

2. On a plate mix together the porridge oats, sesame seeds, low sodium salt and black pepper.

3. Dip each salmon portion in the oat mixture and press all over so that the oats coat the fish evenly.

4. Brush a non-stick frying pan or griddle with a little olive oil (or use an oil spray), heat then add the salmon. Cook over a moderate heat for 3 minutes on each side, covering with a lid. The salmon should be light brown and crispy on the outside. Serve with the lemon wedges.

Health
Salmon is a concentrated source of omega-3 fatty acids, which help reduce the risk of heart attacks and stroke, as well as benefiting the skin, reducing the appearance of wrinkles and also helping control blood pressure. Oats provide soluble fibre, which helps lower cholesterol levels and promote a healthy digestive tract.

INDEX

air pollution 68
alcohol 40
antioxidants 27–9
aromatherapy 61
artificial additives 42
avocado and walnut salad 97
ayurveda 63

Bean, Anita 8
beans
bean provencal with black olives 116
beans, lentils and peas 34–5
bio-yoghurt with banana and honey 89
bloating, reducing 18
blood pressure, lowering 19
breakfast 51, 82–9
breathing 58–9

caffeine 39–40
caldo verde 92
carrots
  and almond salad 100
  soup, easy 94
cellulite reduction 17
chewing food 48–9
chicken
  breast of chicken with butternut squash
  mash 122-3
chickpeas

chickpea and red pepper salad with
  walnuts 101
dahl with sweet potatoes and coconut
  120
with spinach and potato 112
chlorine exposure, reducing 70
Chohan, Ko 8
Christmas 9
colds, fewer 18
compote of dried fruit 86

dahl with sweet potatoes and coconut 120
dairy produce and alternatives 36–7, 41
detox
  are you ready to 8–9
  benefits of 13–14, 17–19
  body wrap 7
  foods 31–43
  how it works 14–15
  how often? 75–6
  how to eat after 76–7
  pills 7
  programme 79, 80–1
  science of 21–9
  supplements 27–8
  ten reasons to 17–19
  tips 45–53
  what is? 21–2
  why now? 7–8

your home 71–3
detoxifying system
  colon 25–6
  food to support 24–7
  gut 23–4
  kidneys 23, 25
  liver 23, 24–5
  lungs 24, 27
  lymphatic circulation 24
  skin 24, 26
diet
  check 9, 11, 12–13
  programme, detox 8
  what to eat 31
dinner 108–24
dioxins 66

energy, increase in 18
exercise 56–8

fatty acids, essential 29
fibre-rich foods 50
fish stew with fennel and tomatoes 121–2
fresh food 45
fruit and vegetables 31–3

grains, bread and pasta 33–4
granola with apple 83
grilled red peppers with ricotta and basil
  106

hair, shinier 19
health check 9, 10, 12
herbs, spices and flavourings 38–9
hunger 48, 52, 53

Italian bean soup 96

juices 47
junk food 46

late eating 51
lentil and vegetable dahl with cashew nuts
  111
lunch 53, 90–107

massage 62
meal planning 49
meat and fish 41
meditation 59–60
milk thistle 29
muesli with fresh fruit 85

non-toxic household cleaning products,
  switch to 69
nuts and seeds 35–6

oat muesli with berries 88
oat-crusted salmon with sesame seeds
  124
oils, healthy 37–8
organic food 14, 32–3, 65–6, 71

pasta spirals with grilled vegetables 118
plastic, cutting down on 67–8
porridge with fruit 87
portion control 51
processed food 50

ratatouille 103
raw or lightly cooked food 45–6
recipes 83–124
reflexology 60
rice and broad bean salad with balsamic
    salad 99
rice noodles with vegetables in spiced
    coconut milk 119
risotto with asparagus and peas 115

salads
    char-grilled vegetable salad with rocket
    and pine nuts 98
Greek salad with fennel and mint 104
salt 40–1
sea bass with spring vegetables 105
serenity 19
shopping 53
skin, smoother 19
sleep 52
snacks 38–9, 53
soup 48
    carrot 94
    Italian bean 96
    Mediterranean summer vegetable 93

spicy lentil 95
spaghetti with fresh tomatoes and basil
    110
spiced quinoa pilaff 109
spicy lentil soup 95
stress, busting 56

tea, fruit and herbal 47–8
toasted pineapple with peaches 84
tofu and mushrooms kebabs 114
toxins
    how the body eliminates 22–4
    what are? 22

vegetables
    char-grilled vegetable salad with rocket
    and pine nuts 98
    nest of stir-fried vegetables on rice 113
vegetable curry with black eye beans and
    almonds 117
vegetable stock 91

water 47
weight loss 17
wheat 39
wholegrain rice with roasted peppers,
    tomatoes and mint 102

yoga 57–8

First published in Great Britain in 2007 by
Virgin Books Ltd
Thames Wharf Studios
Rainville Road
London
W6 9HA

A catalogue record for this book is available from the British Library.

ISBN 978 0 75351 119 0

The paper used in this book is a natural, recyclable product made from wood grown in sustainable forests. The manufacturing process conforms to the regulations of the country of origin.

Designed and typeset by Virgin Books Ltd

Printed and bound in Great Britain by The Bath Press Ltd